"Typically when we are overwhelmed with grief, words can only go so far in bringing relief and comfort. These words written by Karla Helbert, however, are the most powerful, useful, insightful and comprehensive that I've ever seen. She is presenting something very special to the world and what she has accomplished is awe-inspiring. Ms. Helbert has pulled herself up from her own loss, and is thankfully now generously sharing her wisdom. I hope that you don't need this book very often in your life, but when you do, it will be your guide and companion to find your way back from a broken heart."

—*Swami Asokananda, President, Integral Yoga Institute of New York*

"Karla Helbert's new book, *Yoga for Grief and Loss*, is much more than its mere title. This book contains within its pages the depth and breadth of grief's nuances, its crevices, its core questions. It is a navigable, shimmering gift that invites the bereaved reader through the darkness of mourning. Practical yet deeply numinous, I recommend Helbert's *Yoga for Grief and Loss* highly; not as a means to heal or cure or overcome grief—rather, this book will help grievers to be with, turn toward, and grow through grief. Few authors have accomplished this with such honesty and grace."

—*Joanne Cacciatore PhD, Professor Arizona State University, Author of* Selah: An Invitation Toward Fully Inhabited Grief, *Founder of The MISS Foundation*

"Finally! In a sea of books on grief that fall dismally short, Karla Helbert skillfully presents a path that companions pain, rather than trying to solve it. Through the lens of yoga, Helbert demonstrates that the true teachings of all spiritual traditions help us find ways to bear the life that's asked of us. We can hold deeply disparate realities—worlds of pain, worlds of comfort—without being forced to choose between the extremes of endless sadness or faux-positivity. *Yoga for Grief and Loss* is part of a new paradigm of books helping to change the way our culture tends to grief."

—*Megan Devine, Licensed Professional Counselor, founder of* Refuge in Grief, *author of* Everything is Not Okay

"This very profound yet practical guide reviews what yoga can offer to someone grieving a loss. Sensitively written and incorporating very current understandings of grief, Karla Helbert's *Yoga for Grief and Loss* offers wisdom and ways to 'adapt, adjust and accommodate' to our new, however unwelcome, reality."

—*Kenneth J. Doka, PhD, Professor, The College of New Rochelle, Senior Consultant, The Hospice Foundation of America*

"In my own grief experiences and sitting with many bereaved students over many years, I have often marveled at grief's capacity to cut through all that is unreal and unimportant and to focus a laser beam of light onto the deepest longings of one's soul, to push aside all the trivialities of everyday life, until all that's left is loving. Karla's book reflects and honors this profound gift of grief.

Unlike so many well-meaning 'Yoga for...' books, this book is not about a prescription to do anything. It is not the disconnected (or misdirected) directive of the therapist or yoga teacher. Rather it is a profound and profoundly loving acknowledgement of grief as an individual process, born out of, and in fact a form of, love.

This book will absolutely become required reading for trainees in my Integrated Movement Therapy training program—it is not only packed with wisdom on yoga, it is truly an invitation for all of us to meet the grieving, and grief itself with a humble sense of spaciousness and allowing. This book is truly a gift."

—*Molly Lannon Kenny, MS-CCC, Vice President of the International Association of Yoga Therapists, founder and director of the Samarya Center in Seattle WA, and developer of Integrated Movement Therapy*

T0299636

"Raja Yoga has been defined as the psychology and philosophy of yoga, two relevant sciences that help us deal with the unknown, such as loss and death. How we deal with them in a way that helps us grieve and find meaning, minimizing suffering and transforming it into wisdom, is the focus of this book.

It is deep and authentic, coming from Karla's personal experience with the loss of her first-born baby, and from her intense study of Raja Yoga, the study of the mind and human behavior, also the foundation of her Integral Yoga teacher training.

I am in awe of her amazing gift of transforming and making available to all, what could be a dry academic study of the ancient texts into a very practical yoga therapy tool that addresses the devastating effects of grief and loss through yoga. Such a refreshing, effective and inspiring approach!"

—Nora Vimala Pozzi, e-RYT500, PRYT, YCaT, Director of Integral Yoga® Center of Richmond and Teacher Training, Yoga Therapist/ Trainer, Raja Yoga Teacher & Senior Faculty at Yogaville.

"As a Board Certified Chaplain working in hospital, hospice, nursing and aging facilities since 1998, I find Karla's book a very useful tool for those in grief. I believe Karla's explanation of the yogic life style and its many paths to be very inclusive, easy to read, study and incorporate into anyone's own life. I congratulate Karla Helbert for presenting to the public this useful tool for dealing with grief from the yogic perspective."

—Swami Sarvaananda, PHD, BCC, PHD in Education Administration, University of Connecticut, 1980, BCC: board certified chaplain, Association of Professional Chaplains, with Chaplaincy training at the University of Virginia Pastoral Care Department, University Medical Center 1998-2001. Hospice of the Piedmont chaplain, 2004-2013, Holy Order of Sannyas, 1977 by Sri Swami Satchidananda

"What a treasure! This is the book that my heart longed for when my own child died and I cast about for something to both acknowledge and bless the transformational fire sweeping through the landscape of my soul. With deeply grounded wisdom, Karla Helbert simultaneously affirms the unmitigated pain of losing someone we love and offers trustworthy tools to help us navigate the wilderness of loss. By engaging the ancient systems of yoga, we are guided to embrace our grief as the sacred state it is and allow ourselves to connect with the Love that 'yokes' us together for all of time."

—Mirabai Starr, Translator of Teresa of Avila and John of the Cross, author of Caravan of No Despair: A Memoir of Loss and Transformation

"Karla Helbert knows the territory of grief. Her deep spiritual understanding, through the philosophy and practice of yoga, is the GPS that helped her navigate the death of her infant son. This is not a book of postures, although they are included. Through the essential teachings of yoga, Helbert's *Yoga for Grief and Loss* shines a light through the clouds of unknowing that follow loss. Let the gift of these teachings be your ultimate guide to welcoming all that arises through bereavement. Read the book and practice the many self-inquiry exercises, meditations, mantras, mudras, yoga breathing exercises and postures, and you will ride the waves of your loss home to who you truly are."

—Amy Weintraub, founder of the LifeForce Yoga Healing Institute, author of Yoga for Depression *and* Yoga Skills for Therapists

Yoga for Grief and Loss

by the same author

Finding Your Own Way to Grieve
A Creative Activity Workbook for Kids and Teens
on the Autism Spectrum
Karla Helbert
ISBN 978 1 84905 922 0
eISBN 978 0 85700 693 6

of related interest

The Essential Guide to Life After Bereavement
Beyond Tomorrow
Judy Carole Kauffmann and Mary Jordan
ISBN 978 1 84905 335 8
eISBN 978 0 85700 669 1

The Supreme Art and Science of Raja and Kriya Yoga
The Ultimate Path to Self-Realisation
Stephen Sturgess
Foreword by Dr. David Frawley
ISBN 978 1 84819 261 4
eISBN 978 0 85701 209 8

Mudras of India
A Comprehensive Guide to the Hand Gestures
of Yoga and Indian Dance
Cain Carroll and Revital Carroll
ISBN 978 1 84819 084 9 Hardback
ISBN 978 1 84819 109 9 Paperback
eISBN 978 0 85701 067 4

Chair Yoga
Seated Exercises for Health and Wellbeing
Edeltraud Rohnfeld
ISBN 978 1 84819 078 8
eISBN 978 0 85701 056 8

YOGA

for Grief and Loss

Poses · Meditation · Devotion · Self-Reflection
Selfless Acts · Ritual

Karla Helbert

Foreword by Chinnamasta Stiles

Photography by D. Randall Blythe,
Brian Brown, Jamie Fueglein and Karla Helbert

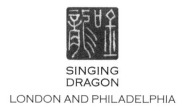

SINGING
DRAGON
LONDON AND PHILADELPHIA

First published in 2016
by Singing Dragon
an imprint of Jessica Kingsley Publishers
73 Collier Street
London N1 9BE, UK
and
400 Market Street, Suite 400
Philadelphia, PA 19106, USA

www.singingdragon.com

Library of Congress Cataloging in Publication Data
Helbert, Karla.
Yoga for grief and loss : poses, meditation, devotion, self-reflection, selfless
acts, ritual / Karla Helbert ; foreword by Chinnamasta Stiles ; photography
by D. Randall Blythe, Brian Brown, Jamie Fueglein and Karla Helbert.
pages cm
Includes bibliographical references and index.
ISBN 978-1-84819-204-1 (alk. paper)
1. Grief therapy. 2. Yoga. I. Title.
RC455.4.L67H45 2016
615.8'2--dc23
2015016603

British Library Cataloguing in Publication Data
A CIP catalogue record for this book is available from the British Library

ISBN 978 1 84819 204 1
eISBN 978 0 85701 163 3

Printed and bound in Great Britain

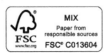

This Book is Dedicated

To my daughter Lula Francys Helbert Fueglein. May your path always be illuminated. I love you more than you will ever know.

And to all who walk the path of grief, this book is dedicated to you and to the memory, the light and the love of your beloveds.

Contents

Foreword

Death is intimate, sacred and secretive. Learning how to live and how to die are equally important to a yogi. We are here in the physical body to live life fully, embracing all joyful and challenging experiences as a sacred weaving of life. Embracing joy is easy; living life gracefully while facing illness or grieving death are not as readily taught and accepted as an integral part of life.

How can you learn step by step to be with yourself while feeling utterly lost, despondent and consumed by pain? What can you do if you have tried everything possible to change your circumstances in life without result and you feel pushed to the point where life loses its meaning?

Grieving the death of a beloved is a personal and unknown journey. A personal relationship with the Self guides you from the heart how to live your life beyond death. With practice that relationship grows on you and is the sacred infinite lap that is always there when you fall apart. It is my personal experience that my beloved has never left me. The sadhana of love we practiced in the physical did not change. It transformed in the formless and showered me with the experience that love is stronger than death. The moment he let go of the last breath, he withdrew himself within me, merged into One. That is where we continue to dance.

This is where worldly life meets the spiritual heart of yoga. Each worldly experience leads you back to the Inner Heart revealing Truth, and the Guidance revealed within the heart leads you back into the world. Where else can you turn but inward seeking the Source of Infinite Love that is always there no matter what the insurmountable pain is you experience in life?

The classical yoga practices are the Source of Serenity, beyond the physical, emotional and mental disturbances. They lead you from darkness to light, gradually, step by step. Life and death become a learning field, revealing when it is appropriate to act, when you have to surrender and how to meet the middle path of wisdom as your friend for life. Worldly life and Spirit life become like a dance of the lover and the beloved. When they gently move closer to one another, spontaneously they merge no longer experiencing separation.

> The seen has the qualities of luminosity, activity and stability. It is embodied through the elements and the sense organs. It exists for the dual purpose of sensory enjoyment and liberation of the Self. (Yoga Sutras of Patanjali, Chapter II Sutra 18, as interpreted by Mukunda Stiles)

You can learn how to be with and move through pain and accept the inevitable while simultaneously experiencing that Spirit is always there. That is the secret being revealed through yoga practices, wisdom scriptures, and the Truth being embodied by wise teachers. The wisdom teacher is there to give the example of a state of serenity no matter what the circumstances are. The teacher holds the space for you to be authentic with your feelings and guide you beyond the mind into a state of infinite love. The classical scriptures are "the body of God." They are the nurturing foods for body, mind and soul that help you carve your life path, while living and loving it fully.

The outer teacher needs to live and share from a place of direct experience, integrity and love. The lessons Karla received through the death of her young child have become lived experiences, and it's from that Source that she shares the yoga practices that supported her. Karla is reaching out and holding hands with you through this book so you may meet your unique path of health and healing, and connect deeply to the purpose in your life.

May many be soothed and nourished by the Divine Mother love that has created this book.

With great respect and love,

Chinnamasta Stiles
Director Yoga Therapy Center &
Shiva Shakti Loka in San Francisco, CA

Acknowledgments

I would like to express gratitude to the Divine. To the Great Mother in all Your forms, source of life, love and creativity, I bow with thankfulness and love.

To my teachers who have been many. Especially to Nora Vimala Pozzi, my first yoga teacher, guide and mentor. Thank you for everything you gave and continue to give. To Gurudev, Swami Satchidananda, without whom the teachings of Integral Yoga® would not exist. To Mukunda and Chinnamasta Stiles, whose work and relationship has been such an inspiration to me throughout the writing of this book. With great respect and love, I honor you both. To Molly Lannon Kenny whose inspiration and guidance brought me so much. To Joanne Kyouji Cacciatore—friend, soul-sister, mentor—thank you. No words can ever be enough.

To my husband, Jamie, for your love, your friendship, for your continued support and unfailing commitment to me, to our family and to my work in this world. Thank you for everything.

Thank you Mark and Karrie Morton for your support, love and hospitality. Randy Blythe and Brian Brown, thank you for your photographic talents, your Karma yoga gifts to this work. Thank you to all the asana models— Kerri Kaveri Helsley, Lydia Nitya Griffith, Jennifer Smith, Sarah Thacker, Nitika Collins-Achalam, Leslie Lytle, Meredith McGlohan-Fotovat. Your spirits shine bright.

To all bereaved who have honored me with the sharing of your stories, your hearts and your beloveds. Thank you so much, you and your loved ones are all my teachers.

Om Shanti.

Chapter 1

Why Yoga for Grief

This is whole. That is whole. When a portion of
wholeness is removed, what remains is whole.

The Purnamadah, Invocatory verse of the *Ishavasya Upanishad*

I n Sanskrit, the historical and liturgical Indic language in which the ancient texts and teachings of yoga are written, the word *yoga* means "union." The Sanskrit word is *yog* with the short *a* sound occurring naturally after the *g*. Said aloud, the word reflects its true meaning, "to yoke": to bind, to join, to unify. The union of yoga describes unification, the yoking together of mind, body and spirit. A great part of this union, and one of the benefits of yoga, is the increased ability of the practitioner to become more aware of the workings of both mind and body and of the intimate connection between the two. Our thoughts create our feelings, and our bodies experience, hold and express these feelings. The more aware we become of this connection, the better able we are to manage, tolerate and even change our thoughts and our feeling states.

Beyond even this is the ultimate and true goal of yoga, which is union. It is the realization that we are connected to, unified with, and *one* with something greater than ourselves. Some conceive of this something greater as God, the Universe, Spirit, the Divine, our Higher Selves, the True Self; there are many names and ways to call this Greater Something.

The concept of the true unity of yoga also includes the awareness of unity with all creation, with all human and non-human life forms, with the energies that exist here on our planet, within the cosmos and beyond. Whether we know it, recognize it or believe it, this is the goal and the ultimate result of the diligent practice of yoga.

Yoga is a path, a way of life, and a way of being that can help us to understand and realize, "to make real," this truth, or Truth: We are part of, connected to, and one with something greater than that which we perceive as our individual selves. The unity of yoga is the realization and remembering of what so many of us have forgotten: All aspects of self—body, mind and spirit—have never been removed from Oneness. We are, and have always been, united and whole. We have simply forgotten this union. We may spend hours, days, months, years, or even lifetimes in a place of forgetfulness of our natural and true state of wholeness. Yoga helps us to remember.

The experience of deep and profound grief tops the list of things that contribute to our forgetting. At some point all of us will experience grief due to the death of someone we love. If we live long enough, and love deeply enough, we will experience this kind of grief more than once. Death is part of life. Everything that lives must die. Plants die, animals die, people die. It is a fact of life that life comes to an end. Death and life are inseparable. One does not exist without the other.

Our conception of death and dying is very individual, shaped and often limited by what we have seen and learned from family, friends, teachers, preachers, therapists, books, media and all of the cultural influences that surround us. How we experience grief is also very individual. Many people do not consciously acknowledge the reality that they will experience the deaths of people they know and love, any more than they consciously acknowledge the reality that each and every one of us, personally, will one day die.

There are whole schools of psychology and philosophy that tell us that every neurosis and anxiety we humans experience is based in the unacknowledged fear and unavoidable certainty of our own deaths. Much of the angst we experience in day-to-day life is rooted in the fear of not only the cessation of our existence as living human beings, but in perceived fears of the process of change, of growing older, becoming infirm, senile, powerless and ultimately non-existent. We are also afraid of pain. We are afraid of being alone, of being disconnected from all that we know. We are afraid those we leave behind will forget us, or that it will not matter whether we existed at all. This is untrue but we don't know it, because we have forgotten our Truth.

These fears stem from the non-realization of our own personal power and the forgetting of our essential Oneness. If we really knew that we are perpetually and eternally connected to a power and a force beyond our understanding, if we really knew, like we know that we are sitting right now on this chair or that we are standing on a solid ground, that we do indeed go on, that our existence beyond this known and tangible physical form is unending, that death is no more than another developmental stage that we will move safely through, we would never be afraid. If we truly knew who we really are, we would never be afraid. When it comes to thinking about death and dying, most of us live in various states ranging anywhere from distaste and denial, to uncertainty and insecurity, to states of fear and terror that result all too often in regular attacks of anxiety and even panic.

Many of us also greatly fear the deaths of those we love. Sometimes these fears are acknowledged, sometimes they are not. For some, that fear is so unspeakable, triggering such discomfort and superstition, that thoughts and talk of death are avoided at all costs. Existentialists would say that fear of the deaths of our loved ones is in actuality only thinly disguised fear of our own eventual, inescapable and positively permanent deaths. Fears of aging, of growing old or powerless, are symptoms of this same fear.

I would have agreed that was true before the death of my son Theo. Having lived through his illness and his death, and having since then had the privilege of knowing and working with many others who have experienced the soul-crushing grief that comes when someone you love so much has died, I think differently. I am less afraid of my own death than I was before Theo died. My husband agrees that that he too is less afraid of death. So are multitudes of those who grieve so profound a loss. In order to experience the presence of those beloveds once more, even if for some that belief is a remote possibility and not a guarantee, death would be a small price to pay.

Knowing that our loved ones have braved that undiscovered country makes our own impending journey to those mysterious lands far less fearsome. The prospect of reuniting with those deeply beloved souls is so beautifully inviting that our own deaths can be anticipated without alarm or apprehension. A force of love and longing, so deep and wide that it holds the power to negate the fear of death, is a powerful thing. I don't wish for pain and I hope my death is peaceful and free of trauma, and the thought of leaving behind my daughter, my husband or my parents makes me feel great concern for them. However, those things aside, I can say that in my heart, I do indeed look forward to a day when, after shaking off of this mortal coil, I might be reunited with my beloved firstborn child. This doesn't make me—or anyone else who feels the same—suicidal or crazy; it makes us normal people in deep grief, who long for a day when we might once again fully experience the presence, instead of the protracted and painful absence of our beloveds.

Yoga teaches us that reunification is not a distant dream or imagined hope. It teaches and shows us that we are already unified; that in fact we were never parted. *Unifying* is not a word most grieving people would ever use to describe their experience in or with grief. This is why I am writing this book. It has taken nearly a decade for me to approach this place in my own grief journey. I am, in the writing of this book, steeping myself in the love of my child, in fearlessness of my grief, in my personal *sadhana* (practice), embracing my *dharma* (path or life's work), and stepping out in faith that I am not always completely sure I have.

While much of what you read here of my personal story surrounds the death of my child, because that is my direct experience of my own deepest grief, this book is not about grief following the death of a child. This book is about grief due to death of those we love. It is also about other kinds of loss. Loss occurs across a lifetime in many different forms; it is not always about physical death. Grief is the experience we have when we lose something precious to us no matter what that something precious may be. This book is about learning a different way of being with grief and loss as part of a full and wholehearted life.

Just as grief is not one way or one thing, neither is yoga one thing nor one way. There are multiple yogic paths. Yet all paths of yoga lead to the same place, to the space and place where we recognize our essential wholeness. Yoga allows us to see all the various pieces and parts of ourselves as unified and to recognize that we were never really separate in the first place. It helps us to remember and to re-member those parts of us that we forgot were One. Yoga helps us to realize and remember that we were never separate and can never be separate, from ourselves, from our loved ones, from all of humanity, from our planet, from Spirit, or from God; howsoever you experience God, Truth, the Universe, Spirit, the Divine.

Yoga is not a religion. Yoga can help us to rise above religious confines and aspects of dogma or religiosity that we may recognize as divisive and which no longer serve us. Yoga can also support and augment any religion you may follow, allowing you to go deeper into your own chosen path. Yoga is a spiritual practice, whether we practice it for spiritual purposes or not. The goal of yoga is unification of our own body, mind and spirit with the wholeness of Universal Spirit. Carl Jung, the great Swiss psychiatrist, founder of analytical psychology, father of archetypes and the theory of our collective unconscious, is said to have had a plaque above his doorway inscribed, Vocatus Atque Non Vocatus Deus Aderit from the Latin, meaning "Bidden or unbidden, God is present." Yoga reflects and reveals that truth.

The tradition and school of Integral Yoga®, in which I was first trained as a yoga teacher, and whose founder and guru Swami Satchidananda's teachings I follow, is dedicated to the principle that "Truth is One, Paths are Many." The teachings of my yoga training helped me through my son's diagnosis of a brain tumor, his illness, and his death with more equanimity, peace and, probably, sanity, than I could have done solely on my own. It has been those same teachings that have helped bring me back to a place where my body, mind and spirit can be unified. Grief makes it very hard to see this truth. Grief can in fact smash that particular belief to smithereens. Yoga can help bring us back.

Grief impacts every aspect of our being. It affects us physically, mentally, cognitively, emotionally, spiritually and philosophically, in every aspect of body, mind and spirit. Yoga and its various branches can support the bereaved in being with and moving through acute and long-term effects of grief in each of these areas. The practice of yoga addresses self-care, helps to integrate the experience of loss, and supports feelings of connection and relationship with loved ones who have died. Just as grief is an experience that affects us physically, mentally, emotionally, cognitively and spiritually, yoga sustains and strengthens us in all of those same areas. Where grief can separate and destroy, yoga unifies and creates.

Western culture and society is very uncomfortable with death and grief. After a loved one dies, society wants us to go pretty quickly back to our pre-grief habits, our routines, our level of functioning, our activities; in general, back to who we were before we were suffused with grief. This is also true generally of non-death losses. There is an expectation, sometimes unspoken, sometimes implied, sometimes spoken very loudly, that the bereaved need to "move on," to "get back to normal," "get over it." You need to "say goodbye," to "put this behind you" and "get back to life." The bereaved hear and intuit all manner of expressions that tell them their experience of grief needs to come to an end and things need to get back to the way they were: back to so-called normal. Friends, family, doctors, co-workers, bosses and clergy often give explicit and implicit messages to *do* something; take a pill, go see somebody, get past it, rise above it, let it go. Grieving people are often encouraged, nudged or pushed to be *doing* something instead of being allowed to simply be just where they are in grief.

Or, if not openly encouraged to do something to fix this, then for God's sake, stop being so *overt* about it. Hide it, stop talking about it and quit making everyone else so upset and discomfited. While these messages may be given out of love and concern, they serve only those who are made so desperately uncomfortable with grief and grief's ever-present reminder of death. They often simply want to stop the discomfort of their own feelings, thoughts and fears related to grief, and of death, though they don't always know this. They also want to relieve the distress of seeing someone they care for in so much pain. Many people will spout painful platitudes, offer clichéd commentary and make unsolicited suggestions that they hope will make the bereaved and themselves feel better, and ultimately help to "fix" the problem. But grief cannot be fixed, and those kinds of behaviors from others rarely, if ever, help a bereaved person feel better, but frequently do cause a grieving person to feel even worse. This is not true for everyone, of course. Everyone handles death and grief and the pain that surrounds those things differently.

Overwhelmingly, even with their own fear and discomfort, whether conscious or subconscious, most people who love a bereaved person really do want to encourage, support and help that person move on, to be happy again, to heal. That doesn't sound so bad. But when you're in a place where you don't believe you can heal, and maybe you don't even want to, or perhaps you have no idea how you might begin to heal, and everyone else seems to want you to do just that, but you just cannot seem to do so, the result is simply more pain.

Often the impulse is to push back, out of anger or frustration at feeling completely misunderstood, at having been made to feel, intentionally or not, that there is something wrong with you if you're not "doing better." While this is not a scientifically studied phenomenon, I often hear that bereaved people begin feeling a pushback from others to be better after about a three-month period. There seems to exist an idea that a grieving and bereaved person should go back to normal after about a quarter of a year, or at least be "doing better," which usually means behaving more or very much like you did before death and loss came. This is painful and baffling to a grieving person who can no more change the pain of grief than they can change the weather.

Another reaction on the grieving person's part may be to withdraw. You may begin to feel or believe that you are weak, depressed or abnormal, because the message is that you are supposed to be "healing," but somehow you just aren't. You can't even imagine what "healing" would look like. And what you are feeling is so intensely painful and raw that you can't imagine that anyone can understand or fathom what you are going through. You may even try to pretend that you are "doing better," hiding, dampening or covering your deeply felt pain, fear, anger, confusion, weariness and exhaustion. This is so unfair to those living in deep grief as it creates more pain along with shame, embarrassment and fear that they are grieving "wrongly," or that there is something deeply wrong with them since they are not "healing" appropriately or in a timely fashion.

There are several problems with trying to help someone heal from grief. The metaphor of healing can cause more pain and suffering because of what healing means and how we think about healing. Thoughts and ideas about healing inherently include thoughts and ideas about non-healing. Thoughts of illness, sickness, brokenness and/or symptoms that need to be eradicated or controlled because they do not belong in a healthy mind or body are present in a dynamic that presumes ideas of so-called "healthy" as fundamentally opposite to a known and societally understood state of so-called "grief." Grieving people are not sick or broken. Grief is a normal and healthy response to the death of a loved one. Sometimes grief may make us feel as if we are broken, but we are not broken.

Another problem that is not really a problem, per se, is that the person may not want to heal. She or he may not feel that they need to heal. She may not believe that she *can* heal. Many bereaved fear or dislike the idea of healing as it seems to imply "getting over" their beloved dead as one would get over a bad cold. Healing also seems to include "moving on," the idea of which can feel like leaving the beloved behind. Grief is a form of love. If we do not love, we do not grieve. Often the thought of healing, giving up or having grief removed can cause the same sort of reaction as the thought of giving up our love. Inconceivable.

Yoga is a very healing practice, and can bring healing when and where healing is needed. While grief itself does not need to be healed, in grief there may be aspects of the body, mind and spirit that can and should be healed: trauma of all kinds, physical wounds where they exist, damaged relationships, unhealthy, painful patterns of relating, thinking or being in the world. However, for grief itself, yoga allows for and gives us the means and ways to be in grief and to learn to grow our lives with the experience. Yoga teaches us how to hold seemingly opposing thoughts, ideas and experiences together at the same time. We can be in grief and live a wholehearted, connected life at the same time.

During my yoga teacher training, my teacher Vimala often repeated another of Sri Swami Satchidananda's sayings, "Adapt, adjust, accommodate." It is a phrase I have never forgotten. In grief, the abilities to adapt, adjust and accommodate are invaluable. The experience of life-changing grief is nothing anyone wants or chooses. Knowing that we cannot change reality, we are faced with the task of making our lives conform to a brand new and wholly undesirable normal. However, being able to adapt to change, sometimes almost immediately, particularly for those blindsided by traumatic grief; cultivating the ability to adjust to new realities; learning to accommodate heretofore never dreamed of circumstances, can be quite useful, to say the least.

In our culture, the bereaved are asked implicitly and explicitly to put away pain, experiences, remembrances, treasured pictures of loved ones and even tears. I regularly ask in support groups that no one give a tissue to a tearful person. If a crying person wants one, he or she can get one for themselves, they are readily available. So often when we are crying and someone gives us a tissue, the message is "You're making me uncomfortable, I don't like to see you in pain, this is not the time, big girls/ boys don't cry, clean yourself up—dry your tears." Even if the tissue giver does not overtly mean any of those things, the message is often undeniably to *do* something other than just go ahead and cry.

We often feel shame and guilt in carrying grief. At about three weeks post-funeral we begin to feel unwelcome and unable to openly mourn or express our experience of grief. When we speak of our beloveds and a hush falls across the room, we begin to feel self-conscious. When others say careless things that trigger deep pain or cause us to feel that everyone else has forgotten the memory of the one we hold so dearly, we feel angry, ashamed, or both. When professionals routinely hand out diagnoses of major depressive disorder, anxiety and panic disorders, post-traumatic stress disorder, or physical illnesses and conditions, which are codified and specified and include time limits on how long we are supposed to grieve, we start to believe that there must be something wrong with us. When we are given pills, told to take this, see someone, go here, do this, do that, but don't put it out here in public where we can all see it, we feel even more hurt, lost, confused and alone than we already did. These things are overwhelmingly wrongheaded.

Western society and its medicine focuses on finding and fixing problems, curing and thereby healing a set of symptoms with the objective of getting the afflicted person back to pre-morbid functioning. Grief is overwhelmingly seen and treated as a problem rather than a natural, normal and healthy state of being and feeling that occurs with loss. When we experience loss, we experience grief. It is a normal and natural response. This is what happens. There is no ability or need to fix anything, no ability or need to change anything. We may wish we could change it, we may feel the need to change it, but truly we cannot really change anything.

Grieving people are rarely allowed or encouraged to simply be, to feel what they feeling. Yoga, however, asks us again and again to simply be with what is, with compassion toward ourselves and others, being exactly where and how we are in the present moment. It encourages, allows and supports us in being exactly how and where we are, while at the same time giving us tools, support and space in which to adapt, adjust and accommodate who and where we are now that grief has visited a new and unwanted reality upon our lives.

I often tell those in grief who come to me for help and support that I believe there are two main tasks to manage. They are not easy tasks, and there may be many layers and facets to finding our way through them. The first is that we have to figure out how to have a relationship with someone who is no longer here with us on this physical plane. This is difficult because even if we are fortunate enough to believe and trust that our loved ones are safe, that they are okay, we still have to face life without them.

The way we interact with the people and animals and things we love is predominantly physical. Everything we experience in this world we experience with our physical senses. We see them with our eyes, hear them with our ears, speak to them with our voices knowing they hear us in return, we touch and hold them, we gesture and send messages with our physical bodies, we intimately know their scent, their touch, their presence in our lives in a physical way. We exchange communication, love, nurturing and sharing in physical, sensory ways—touches, hugs, words, song, food, gifts, shared experiences, a sunset, a concert, a road trip, the first time our children say our names, roller coaster rides, intimate dinners, love notes, laughter—and when those ways of being in a relationship are gone, the adjustment is excruciatingly difficult and painful. Figuring out how to have a relationship with someone who is not physically here, and never will be again, is incredibly difficult, yet we must, because to not have the relationship is even more difficult. While it is the case that death ends a physical life in a physical body, it does not end a relationship and it never ends love.

The second undertaking is in the consideration of who we are now that this has happened to us. Deep grief fundamentally changes us, and we can never go back to being who we were before. How we feel, after the death of a deeply loved person, about fundamental truths we may once have thought unshakable can shift dramatically. After loss, we may find that things we used to think were important no longer have meaning. Our perspectives on multitudes of things may change. We may no longer subscribe to labels or categorizations for ourselves or others. Deeply held beliefs may be obliterated. We walk around in sometimes fuzzy, sometimes sharp disbelief that this is now our life, this is who we are now. But who is that? Not knowing what that means or how to navigate the changes that come to our deepest selves can be frightening. We can feel completely unmoored.

Yoga can help us in all of these things. The essential teaching of yoga is that we are whole and perfect as we are, in grief, in pain, in what we may perceive as a state of complete deprivation and heartbreak. Yoga teaches us to accept who we are, where we are, how we are right now. Yoga points us toward a knowing that we are more than a grieving person while allowing and supporting our experience in grief. Yoga helps us see ourselves, our world, the universe, our beloved dead differently, in ways that can lead to peace, even within pain. Yoga allows us to be exactly where we are, when we are. Yoga supports us in accepting where we are physically, cognitively, emotionally, mentally, spiritually in this moment—and then in this one, and again in this one, and when it changes, now, in this moment. Yoga teaches that we are whole and perfect just as we are, even if we do not believe it for ourselves.

In addition to helping us, in subtle or overt ways, to remember and realize our wholeness, there are scores of side benefits to practicing yoga. For thousands of years, practitioners and teachers of the physical aspects of yoga have testified and taught that *asana* (physical posture) practice and yogic breathing exercises (*pranayama)* can provide increased strength, flexibility, circulation and overall improvement of major body functions including digestion and elimination, immune system function and regulation of mental and emotional processes. Yoga in all its forms is a powerful stress management tool. Grieving people have difficulty in all of these areas. Yoga can help us to be and to feel more spacious, to feel able to open our hearts, even when they are breaking, and to trust that we can find ourselves stronger and steadier than we believed we could be. It engages our brains in ways that help us to feel more connected, more uplifted and accepting of what is. Yoga is an all-encompassing path that can meet us where we are in grief, grounding us, even as it lifts us up.

What this book does

This book looks chapter by chapter at each path or branch of yoga specifically in relation to grief and how each branch can help meet a grieving person's needs. Each chapter also offers suggestions and practices that can help you to cultivate your own practice of each branch.

No one path of yoga is better than another; they all lead ultimately to the same place. Most yogis practice a combination of different branches, drawing on different techniques and aspects of each. Most people who practice *Hatha* yoga's physical asana also study and practice many aspects of *Raja* yoga and its principles. They may choose to engage in ritual of *Tantra* or *Bhakti*, and almost all yogis at some point utilize the self-inquiry of *Jnana* and contemplate the essence of who we really are. Many yoga practitioners engage in selfless service through the path of *Karma* yoga. Choose whatever aspect or practice of any branch you like, pick what resonates with you or that arouses your curiosity or seems to match your interests and try it out. It is okay to combine and create your own practice. It is okay to combine yogic practices with any other spiritual path you practice. I encourage it. Doing so is an act of creativity. Creation is the antidote to destruction. Not to death, because nothing can change death in our physical world, but creation is most certainly the antidote to the perceived destruction that can be wrought by death and by grief.

As you move through this book, feel free to read and do the suggested practices in order if you like, or skip around, reading where you feel most drawn. You might choose to begin with the Hatha chapter to move your body through *surya namaskar*, the sun salutation, or to learn breathing practices that can help calm the anxious monkey-mind of grief. If you are too tired to move, you might flip to the chapter on Raja to see how you might begin to think differently about how you treat yourself or to learn how to sit quietly with compassion toward yourself, and begin to become better able to tolerate and detach from the swiftly changing thoughts and feeling states that can plague the mind of grief. You may wish to examine the principles of Jnana yoga, the path of knowledge, truth and self-inquiry, to understand and gain insight about yourself and who you truly are. You might open the chapter on Bhakti and see how you may already be a devotee of Love or check out the Tantra chapter to see that you can connect with the Divine in the seemingly mundane, and how this includes our beloved dead. If you can't imagine sitting still or being present in your own body or care about the Divine this moment, you might wish to turn to the chapter on Karma yoga to learn to place your energy into action that can help others. In yoga there is something for everyone at all times and places on the path of grief, which is long and winding.

You'll find the use of Sanskrit throughout this book. Sanskrit is the ancient language first used in the founding and teaching of yoga. If you are not a student or teacher of yoga and don't know much about Sanskrit, that's okay. The meanings of the words will be clear in context and I will always provide the definitions and sometimes the nuances of the words throughout.

I suggest using a journal as you move through this book. It will be a useful place for documenting your experiences with the experiential exercises throughout, as well as for recording your thoughts, fears, hopes and insights through grief and in your yoga practice. Journaling can be incredibly helpful. Writing about how you are feeling and what you are experiencing in grief can be both contemplative and an exercise in expression to release and relieve. You can also use a journal as a way to look back to see how your experience shifts and changes over time. This can be interesting and illuminating as we often feel that we will be stuck forever in one place when we are in deep grief. This is never true. It changes all the time, moment to moment, day to day, year after year.

Journaling exercise

Part 1

Using your journal write down all the symptoms, signs and results of grief that you have experienced or that you have seen or heard of in others. Include as many as you wish or as many as you can think of. It is important to note that you may feel or re-experience some of these as you recall them. Please know that this is okay. No feeling state is permanent and this will pass. This can be as short or elaborate an activity as you wish. You can do it in a group with others, or you can skip it all together. Do what feels right to you. Once it is done, put it aside until you finish part 2.

Part 2

On a separate page write down all the benefits, experiences, results and goals of yoga that you have experienced or that you have heard of from others.

When you have finished both parts of the exercise, compare your two lists. What patterns emerge from these two compilations? How are these lists different and how are they similar? Do the words on your lists contradict each other? Do they overlap? How do you feel after reading the two lists side by side? There is no one right or wrong answer. This exercise is about process, and is about making concrete realizations on how you think and feel by merely looking at what you write.

Chapter 2

Jnana Yoga

The Path of Knowledge

Jnana yoga, pronounced *nya-na*, is the path of knowledge and self-inquiry. It teaches us to look into the truth of who we truly are and what we are experiencing. Though Jnana arose from the Hindu philosophy of non-dualism, or *advaita*, the Sanskrit for "not-two," it is not based on any idea, dogma or system that you must believe before you can practice. Instead, Jnana is based on your own direct experience of yourself, which cannot be taught, given or modeled by anyone else. At its simplest and purest level, Jnana asks that you pose questions to yourself about yourself and your true nature, which lead to the primary and sole question in Jnana yoga: *Who am I?* Jnana teaches that the full realization of who we truly are brings about enlightenment.

We can start the inquiry by asking ourselves questions about our experiences in the world, about what we think or feel, and about the truth of those experiences. Ask yourself questions about your own thoughts, experiences, feelings and motivations, and answer them honestly, on a daily basis. I find this practice a helpful tool for relieving a great deal of suffering for myself and have seen it help many people who come to me because of suffering. We can begin by recognizing that most of the things we tell ourselves are not true. When we can learn how to notice the things we tell ourselves and become clearer about whether those things are true—and often they are not—we become clearer about what is actually and absolutely true for ourselves and in our lives overall. Beyond that, we can become clearer about why we suffer due to our thoughts and the beliefs we carry, and what we tell ourselves about them.

Practicing truth-telling with ourselves can be difficult because we tell ourselves things that are not true so frequently that we usually don't even notice that we do it. I have a bumper sticker on my car that reads, "You don't have to believe everything you think." Not automatically believing everything we think and asking ourselves whether a thought is actually true can help us to be free of ideas, opinions, judgments and beliefs that do not serve us.

How can we know whether something is true? Once we get practiced at noticing what we think and tell ourselves, we get better at allowing our intuition to rise, telling us whether something is true for us. Grief can painfully damage our connection to intuition; it can make us feel so vulnerable and uncertain that we may go for long periods feeling unable to hear our own truth, unable to trust our own inner voices. Yoga can help us learn to trust our intuition again, or even for the first time, as the practice of going inward, practicing mindful inquiry, and noticing what is, right now, over and over, helps us regain the sense of connectedness that is inherent in trusting our intuitive knowing.

Something cannot be called truth if it changes all the time, and thoughts and feelings shift constantly. What you think and tell yourself at any given moment is influenced by so many variables; whether you are hungry, tired, irritated, happy, peaceful, sad, ill or hurt; if you are satisfied, calm, confused, overwhelmed, anticipating, anxious or angry. Since thoughts and feelings can shift so dramatically based on mood or physical state of being, how can they be *truth*? A profound lesson that can be learned in this practice is that you are not your thoughts or your feelings.

In grief, this means that you are not your grief. Grief is also an experience that shifts constantly. You can say you are grieving and this can be true. Even more accurate is to notice the experience, the feelings, and what you are telling yourself in moments of grief and to say "This is grief," rather than, "I am grieving." Rather than equating yourself to a state of being, focus on simply defining the emotion or the state as temporary, not one of permanence. We certainly experience grief in all its manifestations, and for long periods of time, but to identify who you are with your feelings and experiences in grief is not the truth of who you are.

Meditation

Grief in the now

In this experience, you are asked to allow the feelings of grief to be what they are. All who've grieved deeply understand that grief comes in waves, moving in, receding, coming forward and then retreating. You can call up experiences and feelings of grief that you have had in the past or sit with the grief you are carrying now. Inviting feelings of grief to rise and then moving away from them can be extremely difficult in early grief, even frightening. Some who are further down the grief road may feel more comfortable with this experience. You never have to do anything that you do not feel safe doing. It can be hard to understand why in the world anyone would want to purposefully call up feelings of grief if they are not right here right now. However, this practice can give you a sense of control over your own feelings and allow you to see that you can manage intense and difficult feelings.

You may find that purposely creating a safe space and time for practicing your ability to allow grief to rise and to be can help tremendously in managing grief when it comes at other moments. The chaos of grief is unpredictable, particularly early on when it comes fast and hard and without a lot of resting space between what can feel like onslaughts. Creating your own space and time to get to know your grief, and to allow it to be, can release the pressure of grief that can build and spill over into our everyday lives. If it feels too scary, you may not be ready to do it. This is okay. Allow what is to be.

If you wish to practice this meditation, feel free to gather photographs of your loved one, journal entries from times when you were in deep pain, play music that reminds you of your loved one, or simply close your eyes and allow your mind the freedom to cast back to a time and place when your grief was fresh, raw, tender. You probably know exactly the photos, memories, songs, thoughts that can produce your grief. As you remember and see in your mind's eye those events, notice how the thoughts themselves seem to call forth the feelings. The memories and thoughts about the memory occur in the mind; the feelings rise in the body. You may notice feelings centering in the belly, the heart, the lungs, the throat, the solar plexus. Your arms may ache; your head and third eye area between the brows may throb or tighten. Your legs may feel weak, you may feel pulled downward toward the Earth, or you may have the sensation of struggling to find balance.

If you feel ungrounded, place your hands or feet on the ground. You might also try holding a stone in your hands. You may wish to turn to the Hatha chapter and look at the description and photo of child's pose, *balasana* (Figure 7.70, page 292), and take this posture to help you feel comforted and more grounded. Try to take slow, full breaths, with the inhale centered in the diaphragm. If you notice your breath becoming shallow or fast, deepen the breath as much as possible to maintain a sense of calm. Whatever you are feeling, notice. Try to create a space of observation, of witnessing your own experience. These are thoughts and feelings, and they will shift and change.

You might visualize a volume dial or a heat thermostat that you can turn up or down to lessen or increase the intensity of the feeling. If the pain becomes too much, dial it down a bit. When you come to a place that feels allowable, simply permit the feeling to be. Think: *This is grief*.

Take note of where sensations occur in the body, where they are most intense and where they are less concentrated. As you inhale, direct your breath into the place in your body where you feel the most intense sensations. Imagine that the breath moving into that area creates space around the sensations, allowing you more room to breathe and to be, so that you can expand into the awareness of what is. Know that you are safe in this experience. *This is grief*. This is how and where you are experiencing your grief right now in this moment.

Be with this feeling as long as you need to. Notice what posture or positions your body takes. As you breathe in, allow the tender, painful places to become more spacious. Direct compassion toward yourself in this experience of now. As you breathe out, let the breath allow your body to release tension from the space of pain.

This is grief. This is also love. Learning to experience the feelings as they are, allowing them to be what they are, rather than pushing them away, feeling that you should be doing something, taking something, seeing someone, "moving on," doing "better," instead of any of those things, consider what it might be like to simply be with what is present. Think of this: Grief would not exist if not for love. When you consider what you feel in grief as a form of love, does this alter the experience? Does it change your thinking about your grief or how you are experiencing it?

When you are ready to end your grief experience in this moment, dial your intensity control down a bit further with each exhalation. When you are ready, close your eyes, bring your hands, palms together, to your heart center in the hand position of *anjali* mudra (see Figure 2.1).

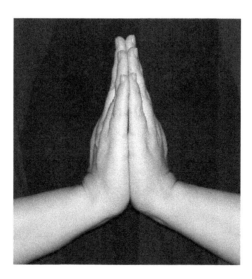

Figure 2.1 Anjali mudra.

In the yogic tradition *mudra* means "attitude," "gesture" or "seal." This generally connotes an energetic or spiritual type of seal. Hand positions are known as *hasta* (hand) mudras. Anjali mudra, also called "prayer position," is extremely common, and is used as a greeting or parting, a gesture of thanks, of respect and devotion, in prayer, and in yoga classes all over the world. Pressing the palms together quiets the brain and creates an energy circuit around and through the body.

When you feel calm and at peace, open your eyes. You may wish to place your hands on the ground, visualizing the Earth beneath, and imagine discharging excess energy, or pain, into the ground, where it can be neutralized and recycled. Send a thank you to the Earth for taking what you are giving.

The greatest tool in Jnana yoga is self-inquiry, the practice of asking questions about ourselves, our experiences and who we are. It is a simple practice, but it is a process. It can be useful to support the practice of self-inquiry with other yogic practices and vice versa. A combination of the various paths of yoga practiced in concert can be very helpful in supporting the practitioner through life and on each person's individual path. Self-inquiry is the primary tool in Jnana yoga for the attainment of self-realization, the realization of the true nature of our mind, body and spirit.

It is a process of examining all of our "I" thoughts and statements, all identifications with our thoughts and feelings, as well as identifications with people and things outside of us. It is as simple as noticing that despite what we may think or feel about things, objects and people around us, we are not those thoughts. What our thoughts reflect are not who we are. We are not our own bodies or even our minds. So then who are we? Who are you? Who am I? This simple question can lead to self-realization and the truth of who we really are. This, however, as in so many facets of life, is often easier said than done. It is simple, but not easy.

An important point about truth-telling through self-inquiry is how to know when something is true. How can we recognize truth? Just because something seems true doesn't make it true. Appearances can be deceiving.

Appearances are based solely on our sensory perception and what we already think we know about something. Our senses can be wrong. Our whole world, how we see things, how we hear things, is experienced through our individual sensory processing. We experience the sky as blue not because the sky is actually blue, but because this is how our eyes experience the occurrence of the kind of light waves that we call blue. The light from the sun appears white, but it is actually made up of all the colors of the rainbow. Because blue light has the shortest and fastest wavelength, we perceive it first. To say "The sky is blue" is actually not a true statement. It only appears to be blue based on our perception. So how can we know what is true?

As we discussed earlier in this chapter, the way that we know what is true is that things that are true do not change. We've established that thoughts and feelings then cannot be called absolute truth because they invariably shift and change. How can we know what things do not change? In grief, the pursuit of truth can be a difficult thing. Nothing feels more true than the desperate pain of grief after the death of a beloved, the sense of absolute destruction of our hearts, minds, lives and all the conceptions we carry of ourselves and who we are. In moments of intense grief and pain, we can feel as though we will never stop hurting and that we will always hurt just like this forever. It can seem unbearable. Then it changes. It shifts, it becomes something else. Again and again this happens.

After the devastation of death or other deep losses that cause grief, the central Jnana question "Who am I?" can be incredibly helpful in supporting movement toward the recollection of original wholeness, even when we don't believe we can ever be whole again. No person who knows the experience of deep grief would argue with the observation that we are changed, we are not who we were before the loss. So, then, who are we?

Questioning can begin with the various connective and relative identities and labels that we apply according to society and our world, our thoughts about the world, our places in it. In so many ways when the life of a deeply beloved person has ended, the bereaved often question whether our roles can still be fulfilled. Without the other, are we still mother, father, husband, wife, sister, brother, grandparent, friend? I say, absolutely, yes. We don't stop being who we are to others and they don't stop being who they are to us just because of death, whether we are the deceased or the living. That bereaved people are encouraged to "say goodbye," find "closure," or subscribe to any other thing that indicates finality of relationship or of the person makes no real sense insofar as the relationship goes. Saying goodbye is unnecessary and serves only to increase pain, confusion and isolation. Intuitively, many grieving and bereaved continue to maintain and seek out bonds with their beloved dead, despite societal or familial disapproval. Moving beyond the label of who we are to those we love, which can never truly describe the depth and strength of the bond of love, we can continue to ask, "Who am I?"

If we think about this question, we can pretty easily cross our bodies off the list of who we are. Merely the way we speak about our bodies tells us that we are not our bodies. Our bodies are always changing from birth to puberty to middle age to old age, all the way to death. They change through illness and injury, childbirth and breastfeeding, by accident and addiction, through rehabilitation and recuperation. The body we woke up with this morning is not the body that will lie down to sleep this night. We most likely have more limited range of motion immediately upon waking, and are more flexible at night after moving around during the day, or we may feel tired and achy after a long day of repetitive movement. We gain weight, we lose weight, we get taller as we grow and shorter as we age, our cartilage flattening, fluid in our spinal discs becoming compressed, muscle mass shifting over time. Our faces become lined after years of moving the muscles in the same ways through smiling, laughing, eye-rolling, squinting or puzzling over questions both shallow and deep. Our bodies change so much, yet we are so often identified with them.

Imagine calling over to your neighbor to borrow sugar. Your body takes you there. When you arrive, your neighbor may ask how you are doing and you might tell her how you hurt your back the other day when you were doing yard work, or that you had a great time getting your nails done, or she may comment on your new haircut. When we talk about ourselves we say "me" and "I." When we talk about our bodies, we use the possessive, "mine." Possessions come and go and are not truths. Possessions are things that we use or enjoy or hold for a time. If our bodies are possessions, we cannot be our bodies.

We are also not our personalities, which are changing all the time and are based on patterns of thinking, feelings and attitudes, as well as all sorts of behaviors, all of which are changeable. Any of these may be deeply ingrained, but are also mutable and much of what we call our personality is based on past experiences we may not even remember. Aspects of our personality may be present at birth. Ask any parent: No baby comes into the world without a personality. But are the glimmers of character, humor or temperament that come with us into the world who we truly are?

Can we be defined by roles we play, groups we belong to, professional titles, jobs we do or beliefs we hold? If you say you are Christian, can you be compared to all other Christians? If you decided you wanted to convert to Buddhism or to Judaism, would you still be you? If you have devoted your life to a career that has defined you, and you change jobs or retire, are you still you even though you don't do that job anymore? Even our names cannot be who we are, because of course, as Shakespeare told us, a rose by any other name would smell as sweet. What about those who change names for marriage, professional or other personal reasons? Most of us didn't even choose our own names; they were given to us by our parents or someone else who most likely didn't even know us yet, or knew very little about us and nothing of who we would become. When we think about these things we can conclude that we are not our possessions, our labels, our roles, our bodies, our professions, our personalities or our names.

So who are you? Who am I?

Journaling exercise: Who am I?

This exercise is gratefully adapted with permission from the book *Your Mythic Journey: Finding Meaning in Your Life through Writing and Storytelling*, by Sam Keen and Anne Valley-Fox.

Think about all the various ways you identify yourself in the world and in your mind. Make a list of the ten words that you feel describe you the best. The words (or phrases) might be titles, functions, roles, feelings, activities, qualities—for example, teacher, compassionate, silly, construction worker, lawyer, brewer of craft beer, healer, artist, student, secretary of state, mother, intelligent, moody, yogi, runner, hipster, open to new experiences.

If you wish to do this activity, please stop here and make your list of ten words before moving forward. Complete each section before moving on to the next. Not knowing what comes next better allows the fullness of this activity to make an impact.

Once you have written your ten words, rank them in order of importance.

Next, cross them out, giving them up one by one until you are left with what you feel is the single most important distinguishing facet of your identity.

As you cross out these identifications you may feel a sense of loss, to deeper or lesser degrees depending on your attachment to each identification and depending on your own history of experience with loss. Allow the feelings and your experience to be as they are. What thoughts occur? What feelings do your thoughts give rise to? Where do you feel what you are feeling? What happens in your body as you have these feelings? What other thoughts and subsequent feelings arise? Simply notice without judgment, as much as possible. Make notes in your journal of your observations.

In the center of a separate piece of paper, write the remaining, most important and distinguishing word or phrase. Contemplate what it means to be this. How is this aspect of your identity truly you? *Is* it truly you? Is there any way that this aspect of you could, would or might be given up, changed, made different, released, liberated or obliterated? Is it a truly permanent state? Is it true? With all your identifications dissolved, who are you?

Write the words, "Who am I?" on another piece of paper.

Under these write, "I AM."

Meditation on I AM

You may also choose to substitute I AM with the Sanskrit phrases SO HUM, meaning *I am that*, or AHAM which means, simply, *I am*.

Sit comfortably in a chair or on the floor. Allow your spine to be straight but not stiff. Place your hands in anjali mudra (see Figure 2.1), or take the jnana hand mudra (see Figure 2.2). To take this mudra, bring the thumb and index finger together so they lightly touch. The remaining fingers are extended and relaxed. Do this with each hand and allow the palms to face up. You may also simply allow your hands to be open, palms up, on your thighs, knees or in your lap.

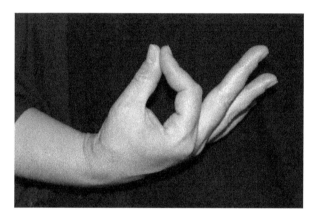

Figure 2.2 Jnana mudra.

Holding the words *I am* softly in your mind, allow and imagine the heart space to be open. Notice that your sitting bones feel solid and secure; extending from the base of the pelvis, these are the two horseshoe shaped bones under the flesh of the buttocks that we literally sit upon. Closing your eyes, imagine your eyeballs dropping backward and down, relaxing and softening toward your throat and your heart. Allow your breathing to become soft and regular.

Allow the words *I AM* to leave your mind and imagine or envision them above your head. Imagine them growing larger and glowing softly with white light. Notice how they are formed. Are they rounded or scripted, flowing or geometric? Notice how they appear to you in your mind's eye. Allow them to be what they are. Allow them to change if they wish to change.

Imagine a circle of light surrounding the words as well as your head. As you breathe in and out imagine the words growing and expanding with their light encasing your entire body in warmth, protection and love. As you inhale, think *I...*

As you exhale, think *AM.*

I...AM.

As you breathe in, imagine that you are directing the energy and warmth of your breath into the space between your eyebrows and imagine *I AM* floating there. Breathe in and out. On the inhale, think *I*, on the exhale, think *AM.* Imagine the color of indigo or deep violet in that space between your brows. If it seems more appropriate, continue to imagine the clear white light. Sit with *I AM* in the space between the brows. Imagine the space between the brows growing less dense, expanding outward and inward. Feel an opening in that space. Inhaling *I*, exhaling, *AM.* Sit with *I AM* resonating in the third eye space as long as you wish.

When you are ready, direct the breath toward the throat area, feel an opening, a spaciousness growing in the throat area, and allow the light of *I AM* to glow softly there. Breathe in *I*, breathe out *AM.* Envision the clear blue light of a summer sky softly radiating from that space. Feel the softness and freedom in the throat's opening and softening.

Direct your breath toward the heart space at the center of your chest. Allow that space to open and soften, expand and fill with the vibration of *I AM*, breathe in *I* and breathe out *AM.* Imagine soft green light, the green of newly sprouted leaves of springtime, to glow in that heart space. You may also choose to imagine a soft pink, a clear white light or any combination of these. Allow the *I AM* to glow in the space of your heart. Notice the fullness and the openness of this space in the front and in the back of the body. Notice the expansion from the sides at the rib cage, opening and expanding. Breathe in *I*, breathe out *AM.*

Direct the breath toward the solar plexus area, just below the sternum, where the ribs meet in the front of the body. Allow the *I AM* energy of the breath to glow like the sun, allow the solar plexus space to expand and open, becoming more spacious, becoming rarefied. Breathe in *I*, breathe out *AM*. Imagine the yellow glow of the sun, radiating warmth all through the torso. Breathe in *I* and breathe out *AM*.

Direct the breath toward the low back between the hips, at the sacrum of the lower back and at the front of the body in the pubic area. Allow that space to open and soften, to become more spacious. Breathe in *I*, breathe out *AM*. Imagine a soft orange glow warming, opening, creating spaciousness throughout the sacral area. Breathe in *I* and breathe out *AM*.

Direct the breath toward the very bottom of the spine and to the soles of the feet. Allow the sitting bones to feel rooted and soft at the same time. Allow the soles of the feet to feel warm, to soften and feel spacious and light. Imagine a deep and vibrant red light glowing at the root and at the soles of the feet, wherever you are attached to the seat or to the Earth. Allow *I AM* to breathe in and out with your body. Breathe in *I*, breathe out *AM*.

Sit with *I AM* as long as you wish.

Go to your journal to write, draw or create any kind of rendering of this meditation experience. Note the feelings you experienced, emotional states, words that floated up in the mind, bodily experiences, physical sensations, visions or imaginings that occurred.

Pain in grief

People do not like to feel pain in general. Even those who appear to seek out pain purposefully, through such practices as tattooing or piercing; those who push their bodies to the absolute limit in stringent athletic pursuit; those who do damage to their bodies internally through overuse, misuse or abuse of substances; those who cut themselves; those who engage in violent fighting or other damaging things, are actually seeking to find or move toward something else that can either help them feel more fulfilled, or to escape something that they perceive as even more painful than the pain that they think are in control of by virtue of inflicting it on themselves. And, of course, pain itself is completely subjective. How I experience pain is not how you experience pain. Human beings in general, though, tend to avoid pain and discomfort and seek out things that are comforting and distracting from pain. Some might call this "avoidance" and this tendency in people can create problems in our lives.

People often avoid the pain of grief by doing all sorts of things, often at the behest of others, sometimes because they don't know what else to do to find solace or relief from the pain. However, it's almost impossible to avoid the pain of grief. Much of this book has to do with not avoiding or escaping or relieving pain, but entering into the pain, even though this may seem counterintuitive. Instead of moving away from the pain, learn to let the pain be what it is, even invite it in, set aside time for it in various ways, move into the pain as much as possible without fear. We can observe, witness and examine the pain as part of the experience we are having. We can note how it changes. We can recognize that, even though it hurts, when we allow it to be what it is, it may not be nearly as frightening as we may have once believed it to be.

When we are in grief, our whole being is affected. We are plunged into chaos, not knowing how we are going to feel from one minute to the next. We might be feeling okay, able to get up, get dressed, maybe go out in the world, get some errands done, engage in life in some way, alongside the surreal comprehension that the rest of the world has not stopped for the death of our beloveds. Life apparently does go on elsewhere, even when we may not want it to.

So, say it's a day when you can get up, get dressed, go out, do some things. There you are in a grocery store aisle, standing in front of his favorite cereal. Thinking about how you need never buy that cereal again. Or you find yourself standing in line at the post office behind a woman holding her sleeping toddler, thinking of how you will never hold your sleeping toddler in any line, anywhere, anytime. The momentary feeling of being okay, functional, able to manage some minor task is gone and you are again plunged into an ocean of grief. A song may come on the radio, the lyrics of which you never considered to be about grief and longing, but suddenly it is all about your pain and your beloved who is missing from your life and you have to pull over to the side of the road because tears have made you blind. These kinds of moments happen over and over again in grief. Rarely do we see them coming. Sometimes we can see them coming, but we can never truly predict how we are going to feel. It is exhausting and often frightening.

Spiritual teachers and sacred texts both ancient and modern tell us in many different ways that the reason we are not at peace right now is not because of our circumstances, but because of what we tell ourselves about our circumstances. We suffer because we want things to be other than what they are. After my son died, it was incredibly difficult for me to read any kind of spiritual teaching or writing. If I tried to look at my circumstances from any perspective than my own bereft state, all I could come up with over and over again was, *Yes, that is all well and good, but my son is dead!* I wondered if the writer of whatever words of wisdom I was reading knew what it felt like to have a dead child, and doubted they would be saying those things if they did.

I remember vividly how I felt when his death and his permanent absence from my life were the first things I thought of every single morning. I would open my eyes from sleep and experience the brief space of time of thinking nothing really, reorienting to the waking state, and then the thought came floating up—*Theo is dead*—and the heaviness settled itself around my heart. Or, sometimes, the thought didn't float, but crashed in, mean and shocking, rushing into my awareness like a blast of freezing air or having the breath knocked out of me. Sometimes it woke me up that way, like an alarm, feeling like a shock to my system. But usually the thought just kind of drifted in, reminding me, as if I needed a reminder: *Psst...hey...your baby is dead... remember?* My heart was seared anew each morning.

I also remember when I noticed that it was no longer my first thought upon waking, and the strange pain that realization brought with it as well. That thought is never the first thing I think when I wake now. His picture is on my nightstand. His sweet face is the first thing I see every morning when

I rise and the last thing I see every night before I switch off the bedside light. But the aching heaviness of that repeated dawning of daily recollection is no longer there. And he is still dead. And it still hurts. But it has changed.

So how can we know what is true? It is still true that my child is dead. That is a fact of my life. It is also true that how I think about it, the feelings I experience around that fact have shifted and changed. So what is true within grief? Looking at spiritual teachings from the perspective of a grieving mother is something altogether different from looking at spiritual teachings from the perspective of who I was before my son's death. After his death I couldn't tolerate reading about spirituality because I knew those things no longer applied to me. But was that true? Not really. It was how I was thinking about it that made the difference. This is not to say that it is easy to change our thoughts, especially the thoughts we have about the deaths of our beloveds and their absence and what that means for the rest of our lives here on Earth. Sometimes simply recognizing that thoughts and feelings will and do shift can be in itself very helpful in a moment of seemingly intolerable pain and longing. You can know that you can bear it in this moment because it will change.

The Buddha taught that life is suffering. That we all suffer in one way or another, over and over until we learn how not to suffer. He also taught that suffering is caused by attachment and if we can learn to live without attachments then we will no longer suffer. It is a risky proposition to tell a mother whose child has just died—or a mother whose child has died last year or five years ago, or ten years ago or twenty—that her suffering is due to her attachment to her child and that if she could just let go of that attachment, she would no longer suffer. If you want to keep your head, or if you want to keep her as a friend, or if you simply don't want to cause her more pain, it might be best not to suggest that she simply release her attachment. This same thinking applies to telling a newly bereaved wife that if she would just let go of her attachment to her husband she would feel better, or telling a child in grief that he should let go of the attachment to his mother or grandmother or the beloved family dog who has just died. It just isn't that easy.

The *Bhagavad Gita*, a sacred Hindu text thousands of years old, speaks of the True Self that never dies. In the book, Lord Krishna speaks to the warrior Arjuna, offering him guidance, showing him the path of Truth. In chapter 2, Arjuna refuses to perform his duties out of grief for those who have died and will die.

> The Lord says to him:
> You grieve for those who should not be grieved for…
> There was never a time when I did not
> exist, nor you, nor anyone…
> Neither will there ever come a time when we cease to be.
> The Self dwells in the house of the body,
> Which passes through childhood, youth and old age.
> So passes the Self at the time of death into another form;
> What is not, has never been; and what is, always is.
> No one can destroy what is everlasting and imperishable.
> The Self is eternal, indestructible and immeasurable.
> The Self is not born and it does not die.
> Unborn, undying, never ceasing, never beginning,
> Deathless, birthless, unchanging forever.
> Not wounded by weapons, nor burned by fire,
> Not dried by the wind, nor wetted by water.
> The Self is not a physical creature.
> There are some who have looked upon the Self
> and understood It, in all Its wonder
> Others speak of It as wonderful beyond their understanding…
> Others have heard of It and understood not a word.
> This Self, which exists in everyone,
> Is invulnerable and deathless, immovable and everlasting.
> Know this truth, and leave all sorrow behind.
>
> Satchidananda (2000)

The Buddha taught similar lessons about what is permanent and impermanent. He did not comment directly on existence after death or even on God, but taught that the Soul, the Self, the Atman, the Divine in each of us, is the only thing we have that is permanent. And those things that are permanent are the only things which are Real or True. Everything that is physical changes: Bodies die, buildings crumble, fortunes disappear, even the very Earth itself can and will eventually be destroyed; the only thing we have that cannot be destroyed is the Soul. It is the only thing that we have that is Real. Everything else is *maya*, or illusion, unreal.

I found a story of the great Tibetan Buddhist master, Marpa, who lived and taught at the beginning of the eleventh century. He was a great teacher and had many disciples. Stories tell of the untimely death of Marpa's son whom he hoped would carry on his work. His students came to visit him after this beloved son's death and were shocked to find their master crying and wailing, deeply mired in grief for his son.

They said, "Master what is wrong?"

Marpa replied, "My son is dead!"

His students said to him, "But Master, have you not taught us that the physical world and everything in it is but an illusion? If this is so, why do you grieve?"

And Marpa said, "Yes, all is illusion—and the death of a child is the greatest illusion of all."

The objective of Jnana yoga is to, through questioning our perceptions and beliefs, and through the use of self-inquiry, come to the absolute Truth about life, and about who we are. Part of the pursuit of Truth is recognizing that *advaita*, non-duality, *not-two*, is the reality and that the idea of dualism, of separateness, is but an illusion. The illusion is a strong one. As the great teacher Marpa shows us in the story above, even a renowned spiritual master struggles with the pain of grief regardless of his teachings and knowledge of the illusory nature of this world. The contemplation of non-duality and the questions themselves can bring us to a place where we can be open to our experience of grief in the moment. If we are one and not-two, then with whom, or what, are we one?

Hinduism, from whose deep roots came the foundation of yogic teachings, is a polytheistic religion. Overarching the conceptions of the hundreds of gods and goddesses that are worshipped and revered in the Hindu system, the belief is that all deities, including those outside the Hindu system, are aspects and manifestations of the One. This One is known as Brahman, the ultimate reality behind, within, surrounding, and permeating everything in the universe, the Supreme Reality behind all illusion. Brahman cannot truly be defined because It is beyond definition, without definition, without boundaries, and without form. Brahman is that from which all else springs. It is the source of everything, all creation, each one of us. A wellspring of pure love, inspiration and abundance. Brahman is known by many names and concepts: the Absolute, Creator, Source, Divine, Great Spirit, Goddess, God, but Its absolute nature is devoid of and beyond any and all religious conceptions, individuations, dogma, mythologies or personifications. Brahman is the ultimate non-duality from which everything in the universe flows and to which we are infinitely connected. And we each, as is everything in creation, are part of the wholeness that is Brahman. Never ending, never beginning. Because we are part of the All, we cannot be separate from the All, nor anything else which is part of the All. Recall once more the etymology of yoga, the word itself meaning *union*. The opening verse of the *Ishavasya Upanishad*, a sacred Vedic text known as the *purnamidah*, translates this way, "From wholeness comes wholeness. When a portion of wholeness is removed that which remains is whole." We can never be separate.

The concept of non-dualism is hard to talk about because in order to talk about it we must use language, which itself cannot be anything other than dualistic. If this is defined as something, then there is something else that this is not. Dualism is the world of concepts, words, opposites, definitions, right and wrong, this or that, up or down, inside or outside, you and me, true and false, male and female, feminine or masculine, white or black, good or bad, approve or disapprove, believe or disbelieve. This could go on day and night. Non-duality is something that goes beyond any concept the mind can construct. Even if we think, feel or believe otherwise, all is wholeness. This is the essence of non-dualism. A state (that is not a state), a place (that is not a place) of pure love, intimacy with all, non-separation from anything, outside of time or even thought. The practices of yoga help us to remember this as our Truth.

The sutras

One of the ways we can begin to experience Jnana yoga is through contemplation and meditation. In yoga, the definition of meditation is the cessation of thoughts. But to simply stop thinking is incredibly difficult for most people. In grief, it can seem impossible to stop our thoughts. Often people, grieving or not grieving, become frustrated with meditation, saying, "I just can't quiet my mind!" I discourage actively *trying* to quiet the mind. It's somewhat like trying not to think about a rhinoceros when someone says, "Don't think about a rhinoceros."

For most of us, the mind thinks almost all the time, it goes on and on and on with its monologues and its chatter, its questions and doubts, the commentary, judgments, predictions and fears, dreams and nightmares. The mind is rarely quiet. This is okay; it's doing its job. If we begin instead with the practice of simply observing the mind and its thoughts, without getting involved and tied up in them, of learning how to simply witness our thoughts, we can come closer to the place of cessation of thought and the gift of slipping into the space of wholeness that is wholly without thought. Once we comprehend we are in a place without thought, we are again thinking. We must let this also be okay. Cultivating the witness, with compassion and kindness toward ourselves, can help us to learn to notice the thoughts and to be less involved in identifying with the thoughts as who we are.

The Yoga Sutras of Patanjali, written sometime between 400 BCE and 200 CE, contain 196 *sutras*—sayings or aphorisms—that describe the science and practice of yoga. Literally the word *sutra* means thread, and is taken from the Sanskrit verbal root *siv*, meaning "to sew." No one truly knows whether Patanjali was one person, or several teachers whose teachings were compiled into one text. Either way, *The Sutras* have become the primary text of yogis everywhere. The 196 sutras discuss every aspect of yoga, they are the threads by which the whole cloth is created and held together. The very beginning of the book contains some of the most important sutras, which in essence are Jnana yoga.

In the first sutra, Patanjali introduces yoga by saying: *Atha yoganusasana.* Now (*atha*), is the instruction of yoga. The most significant thing about this first sutra is the implication of *atha*, now. Now is yoga. It is not simply something that happens on a mat in a studio. This sutra implies the importance of the mindful attention to now, the present moment, and that yoga, the practices, and the union, is now.

In the second sutra, he tells us what yoga is. Sutra 1:2: *Yogas chitta vritti nirodah*: Yoga is the restraint of the modifications of the mind-stuff. *Chitta* translates as "mind-stuff," all aspects of the mind from the yogic perspective including, the ego (*ahamkara*), the intellect (*bhuddi*), the desires (*manas*). *Vritti* means modifications or changes, and is all the goings-on, the shifts, the swings, the drama within all aspects of the mind-stuff, the talking, the contemplating, the chatter, the monkey-mind, the constant commentary, the questioning, the distractions of the senses, ruminating on things of the past, creating illusions of a future that has not yet happened, something shiny over there, something upsetting over here, striving and struggling with all the things we tell ourselves about our circumstances and situations. *Nirodah* is usually translated as restraint, as in curbing, controlling, limiting; sometimes "suppression" as in containment, keeping in check, putting the lid on. We could also see it as the resolution, or quieting of the mind. So, yoga is the quieting down of the chatter of the mind. Sri Swami Satchidananda taught that if only this one sutra was learned, it would be enough, because all the other 195 sutras only explain this one. He also translates in his book, *The Yoga Sutras of Patanjali*, the second sutra to mean, "When you can control the rising of the mind into ripples, you will experience yoga."

The third sutra explains that once the mind is still, *Tada drastuh svarupe vasthanam*, "Then the Seer abides in its True nature." We are the seer, seeing our true selves in our natural, original and eternal state of peace, equanimity and love. When we can quiet the mind, and experience the union of yoga, we are able to see not only our own true nature, but that of others as well, including our beloved dead. In that state of being truly open and awake, we can know that there is no death, no separation. The duality we experience in our mind's workings, in the constructs of thought and language, in the perception of our physical experiences and existence, is all illusion. But as Marpa's story of grieving his son shows, and as all deeply grieving and bereaved people know, grief and the illusion of separateness in death is indeed the greatest, most powerful and believable illusion of all.

The sutras offer a guide, something like a road map through the slings and arrows of seemingly outrageous fortune, to follow in order to help us learn to calm and quiet the mind. Even when we may feel powerless to stop or control its crowded chatter, we can learn to observe its pace and procession, and to continue to cultivate our inner witness. If we can learn to gently, in each new moment of now, observe our thoughts and minds with compassion, we can get better and better at practicing the quieting of the mind. Sometimes we can simply notice what it's saying and doing and choose not to become involved in the thoughts, changing our focus to something else, or when the thoughts are so overwhelming and feel so far outside our purview, such as in intense grief, we can learn to watch what is happening as an observer, as the witness.

In my work with one grieving mother, we spent time talking about and examining her deep suffering, anger and anguish, not only at the death of her beloved infant son, but also with so many other complex feelings that accompany deep grief. On one particular day she described the distress she was feeling at the recent news of her sister's pregnancy. Part of the pain she was experiencing had to do specifically with the fact that this new baby was due on her deceased son's first birthday. This meant, she said, that the child was conceived on or very near the date of her son's death. She felt betrayed, angry and hurt. She recounted a conversation with her mother where her mother could not understand these feelings or her reluctance and disinclination to offer congratulations, or even talk to her sister and brother-in-law. This bereaved mother tried to explain to her own mother how she could not control her feelings. She had tried and failed. She felt angry and betrayed; her mind whirled with accusations, thoughts of betrayal, and disbelief that her sister and the universe itself could be so cruel.

We talked about learning to tolerate and be with the feelings as they are. Much like the weather. We cannot, and it is pointless to try to, control the weather. When there is a gale force storm raging inside our hearts and minds, the notion of control of those feelings can seem preposterous. But we can learn to watch it. To observe and simply be with the feelings, without judgment. This is the place to start. Breathe through the feelings. Let them be what they are. And ultimately, know that they will change. And that we can never control other people's feelings, behavior or responses. When we have feelings about that, we can sit with those as they are as well. Those feelings will also change. No feeling state is permanent.

A month later, her feelings had indeed changed and shifted. She still was not joyous at her sister's pregnancy and she did not look forward to the new baby's birth, but she no longer felt betrayal and ire. She came to a new understanding, recognition that the storm had passed and something else would arise, something different. Not necessarily something sunny and light, or even something better, but different than what she had at one point felt was intolerable. She could clearly see that what she witnessed in the previous storm had indeed passed and that she did survive those dreadful feelings. This helped her to know that she would survive future mind and heart storms as well. Learning to observe and not become absorbed in our thoughts, our *chitta vrittis,* our constantly changing mind-stuff, can help us to avoid the pitfalls Patanjali warns of in the next sutra.

Sutra four, *Vritti sarupyam itaratra,* tells us that when our minds are not quiet, they will assume the forms of the changing mind-stuff (*vritti*), thus distorting our true nature. We think we are our thoughts. I am rageful. I am angry. I am depressed. I am anxious. I am unfit. I am sick. I am stupid. I am ugly. I am inept. I am not enough. We become identified with our thoughts and our bodies and whatever we are telling ourselves about those things. We become walking, talking cases of mistaken identity. Who are we really? Who are we, and who are our beloved dead?

Meditation

Cultivating the witness

I invite you to try the following exercise for at least ten minutes daily. If you can't do ten minutes, try five minutes. If you can't do it for five minutes, ask yourself why you can't find five minutes to spend with yourself watching your thoughts. Think about all the things you spend more than five minutes doing throughout your day. What is rising within that causes you to feel unable to be still? Often when we try to be still, we become suddenly aware of all the internal mind-stuff that we distract ourselves from throughout our conscious hours. When we become still, purposefully withdrawing from the distractions we create day and night, the chatter can become very loud. Our bodies suddenly seem to do everything possible to get our attention: a foot hurts, our back itches, legs become restless, eyeballs can't settle, the body doesn't feel comfortable in its seat. This is all okay. See if you can simply sit with and witness what is happening even for a few minutes.

If it's not possible to sit in stillness, find a way of moving your body without having to think about the movement. Good choices are walking in an open space like a park, running on a track or a treadmill, somewhere you won't have to think about oncoming traffic or other distractions. Try a rocking chair. The gentle movement soothes the body while allowing the mind to be occupied elsewhere. You might also choose to gaze into a crackling fire or at moving water to help soothe and calm the body's impulse to move.

This practice will help you learn to become more aware of the thoughts that come into your mind at any given moment. It can help you become more adept at noticing them when they come at other points throughout your day, when you aren't engaged in practicing meditation. Over time, this practice can help you become better at not getting involved, or hooked into, every thought that might come at any given moment.

There are many different meditation techniques and none is necessarily better than the others; it depends on individual preference. Because the breath is always there with you, I recommend using the breath as a returning point. I suggest labeling the thoughts as they come because it helps you to notice them more easily when they come during non-meditation time, and also because labeling the thoughts as separate from the Self helps to break self-identification with thoughts. You are not your thoughts. You don't have to believe everything you think.

To begin, use a timer so that you don't feel compelled to check the clock. Turn off your phone and other devices that could interrupt you. Find a comfortable spot on a chair or on the floor. If you sit on the floor, you might want to use a cushion or folded blanket to support the sitting bones and help the hips to feel more comfortable. If you choose to sit in a chair, let your feet be flat on the floor. Loosen any tight clothing. Allow your hands to rest in your lap or on your knees in a comfortable position. Allow your spine to be long and tall, but not stiff. Roll your neck from side to side to release tension. Take a few deep, cleansing breaths, focusing on expanding your abdomen. Allow your breathing to return to normal.

Bring your full awareness to your breath. Notice how it feels as it moves in and out of your body, not changing anything, just being with what is and noticing. Allow your attention to remain with your breath, in and out, notice the temperature of the air as it enters your nose, moves down your trachea and into your lungs. Notice that it is warmer and more moist as it gently leaves your body. Notice the movements of your abdomen, your ribs and your chest as your breath moves in and out of your body. Notice the dimension of the breath, how much space it takes up in the body. Notice that there is less space where the in breath turns to exhalation. Notice the pause. Notice where in the body its presence is felt. In and out. Just breathe and notice. Don't change anything, just witness.

Eventually, you will notice that you are no longer aware of your breath. You are thinking about something else. This is okay, and it will happen. When you notice a thought, or an emotion, recognize that you are the observer of the thinking and feeling. You don't have to get involved. You can simply observe. As the thoughts and feelings rise, watch them without trying to control, change, edit or analyze them. You might imagine watching the thoughts appearing and disappearing as if you were alone in a movie theater, seeing your thoughts, feelings, memories playing out their scenes one after the other, or rolling gently up the screen like the credits at the end of a film. If you are more attuned to nature, you might picture watching the thoughts float in and then out of your awareness like clouds across a sky.

For many, the deluge of thought may be far stormier than an image of fluffy clouds floating across an expanse of blue. If your thoughts are more turbulent and chaotic, a more apt representation might be to imagine yourself in the midst of a violent storm, rain pelting your body, thunder and lightning crashing. Visualize this scenario and then imagine yourself finding shelter on a covered porch. Here you are warm and dry. You can sit safely on the front porch swing and calmly watch the storm. If that is still a little too close, go inside and view the downpour from a window. Safe and dry, you can simply watch what is happening, an observer of your own thoughts, as well as any feelings that may rise. As you watch the storm, you may see it shift in its intensity and power.

As you observe, in your place of safety, without judgment and with compassion, simply begin to label your thoughts and emotions as they come and go: Thinking, worrying, planning, doubting, judging, fantasizing, daydreaming, anxiety, fear, impatience, irritation, grief, anxiety—whatever the thought or feeling, give it a label as you continue to watch the flow. If at any time, any thought or feeling becomes too difficult to watch, know that you can shift your attention back to counting your breaths, the sensations of the breath or, if you are moving, to the movement of the body anytime you wish. You can choose where to place your attention. Continue to do this until the timer sounds.

After the timer goes off, take a moment to notice how you are feeling. Take a couple of deep breaths and go on with your day. You may want to write about this experience of witnessing your thoughts in your journal.

What does it mean that you can take a step back and watch the processes of your own mind? How could this be this helpful in grief, in your day to day life? Can you call upon this witness consciousness when you are not practicing meditation?

The witness

As you become more adept at cultivating the witness, you may begin to observe that you become more skilled at witnessing your thought processes and feeling states when you are not practicing your meditation. You may get better in your day-to-day life at noticing the kinds of thoughts your mind churns out and what sorts of things you tell yourself all day long, and how this in turn impacts your mood and how you are feeling. As you practice your meditation, simply noticing and witnessing the progression, the comings and goings of thoughts, feelings and sensations, you become more adept at resting in that witnessing consciousness watching the goings-on within.

In grief, this skill can help us to understand that even though the present moment is painful, it will shift, it will change, and we can be okay. We can breathe and notice the feelings and the thoughts and no matter how intense, we can know that they will pass. They will pass and something new will arise. It may be more or less painful, but we can remain watchful and awake. Remaining open, curious, and observant of what comes can help you learn to adapt, to adjust and to accommodate new feeling states, new thoughts that may arise, anytime, anywhere.

As you continue to observe, you may also begin to notice other sorts of questions arise. If you are witnessing your thoughts and feelings, who is the witness? This witness is the Seer that Patanjali tells of in sutra three. You may also notice that this part of you, the one who witnesses, is amazingly and always calm and peaceful. In his book *The Yoga of Truth* (2007), Peter Marchand writes of the witness consciousness as, "Having neither form nor quality, this you also has no sad or happy past, no hopes or worries about a future, no ideas or opinions to defend, no mood swings, no pain to bear, no hands nor feet. When you can feel the witness to be you, all those just drop off, revealing themselves as separate from you." And, he adds, "Isn't that a relief?" (p.21).

This peace is your true nature which does not and cannot change. It rests always in the pure moment of now, undisturbed, unaffected, serene, and at ease. This is the Seer, the True Self. As mentioned earlier, Buddhism and Hinduism refer to this witnessing consciousness also as the Atman, which is not separate and can never be separate from Brahman, Source, God, Spirit, One, the All. If you and I have a conversation about our witnessing selves— the witness consciousness in you and the witness consciousness in me— and we discuss the liberating realization that our witness consciousness is always peaceful, always in the now, and that our witness consciousness is the unchanging, undying part of us, connected to the never-ending Source of All, how can we fail to notice or wonder at the similarity of our seemingly individual witnesses? Why would it not then follow that each of us has an identical witnessing consciousness, a Seer within which looks out upon all that transpires? Everything we see, sense, think, experience, feel, this witness sees and takes in, calmly, lovingly. As the modern-day philosopher Malcolm Hollick wrote in his work *The Science of Oneness*, "We become open to the experience of this unity only when we recognize at the deepest intuitive level that we do not exist as separate selves" (p.290).

Think of this for a moment: all beings have this witness within. All members and beings of the animal, plant, insect and mineral kingdoms, all the oceans, caverns and mountaintops, have this same witnessing consciousness, seeing, watching, experiencing, observing, feeling, hearing, thinking, being, each in their own individual ways. And since the witness is the only unchanging, *undying* part of who we are, who we have always been, it also follows that our beloved dead exist as well in their unchanging witnessing consciousnesses, somewhere, somehow.

Energy is neither created nor destroyed. All the various reflections of the unchanging, undying Source, are simultaneously experiencing human, animal, plant, mineral and elemental forms of existence through all of creation throughout the universe. We are all connected by that witness which is in each of us, and which is Brahman. Or as some may prefer, Spirit, Source, All, Goddess, God, Creator.

Even if what you read here strikes you as crazy talk, possibly, depending on your personal belief system, bordering on blasphemy, just for a moment, can you suspend disbelief? What if it were true? Or True? Whichever you prefer. Imagine that you are not constrained by disbelief. As Hamlet said to his friend Horatio, I say to you, "There are more things in Heaven and Earth, Horatio, than are dreamt of in your philosophy." We know so very little. To momentarily imagine, even for a brief moment that things are different than we may have previously thought, to suppose that this could be your truth, can broaden the mind to undreamed of vistas of possibility. To do so allows us to say, "I never thought of it that way," and so to envision the possibility of difference. This allows you to ask yourself how things might be different, how can you view circumstances or yourself differently? How might your feelings or your day-to-day interactions with others be altered? Even if you choose not to dive headfirst into this particular philosophy, imagine for a moment that this *could* be your truth. That we *are* all connected, yoked together, parts of a whole that cannot be undone, removed or detached. That we are all united as One; that we are, as yoga teaches, unified, never separate from either our loved ones or from God, our Source.

For now, if you will, think on the Universal Witness, this all-reaching, omnipresent cosmic consciousness, as fact. If you become still and begin to notice, you can sense, perceive and discover the witness within your very own self, without having to imagine. Its presence is fact. This can be your direct experience. Patanjali tells us in sutra 1:7 that one of the sources of right or valid knowledge is our own direct perception, our own personal experience. True insight and knowledge are found through direct perception, logic, reason, and reliable, trustworthy testimony. So, in noticing this witnessing consciousness within, as a direct and personal experience, and comprehending it is a true experience, what then of the experience of all other sentient beings on Earth or in the universe? Peter Marchand asks us:

> Imagine what would happen if you were to add up two of those absolutely formless and fully identical witnesses? Would you end up with two or

would they merge into one? Being formless, would they even need to merge, in order to become one? Does this not mean that the universe has just one witness, looking through many eyes, hearing through billions of ears, tasting through countless tongues…? Are not the many, in essence, just one? (p.24)

I have heard many stories of bereaved people longing for and missing their beloveds, discussing similar concepts of feeling a parallel connection, experiencing things on behalf of, in the stead of, and even alongside their beloved dead, continuing to share in the experience of life with those that are so loved. It is another way of reminding ourselves of that indissoluble connection with those we love who have died.

My husband wrote of our son Theo, and their imagined but deeply experienced connection to each other beautifully and heart-achingly in this way:

I see his head in cloud formations, in the pattern of wood grain on telephone poles, in oil stains, in the black and gray patterns of slate rooftops on distant houses, in the river as it flows over rocks and fallen tree branches, in hubcaps, in streetlamps, in dreams. Sometimes I imagine Theo's head growing right out of my own. It pops up out of my right ventricle, his head with eyes and smile and mohawk. He travels with me, up on my head, looking at all the things I look at, thinking of the things I am thinking, and we are of one head.

Margo, bereaved mother of her 30-year-old son, went on what she called a pilgrimage to the places her son wanted to visit. She took his map and at each stop across the world from Australia's outback to the Space Needle she left a small amount of his ashes. She said of her travels, "He couldn't go these places. I want to go for him. To see the things he wanted to see. Walk the places he wanted to walk. I will walk there for him and leave a piece of him there."

Jnana assists us in coming to a place where we might experience the reality of our non-dual nature, shared with our beloved dead, even for a brief moment, by helping us truly answer the question "Who am I?" in the practice of learning to discriminate between the Seer and what it sees. What the witness witnesses is constantly changing, but the witness remains the same. It is the only part of us that does not change. Our environments change, our thoughts and our moods shift and change, our bodies and roles and identifications shift and change, appear and disappear. The witness, which sees all of this, is never changing. Once the witness, the Seer, the Self, is free from all external associations it can shine forth. Once we can see this truth, that who we are is free from all the chatter, we can watch the mind-stuff come and go, form and dissipate, resting in the knowledge of our True Selves, always connected with our beloveds and with all of creation, existing in pure consciousness and peacefulness.

Meditation

Breathing in the ultimate reality

Another practice that can be helpful in allowing your inner wisdom to rise is to sit quietly, noticing the breath move in and out of your body. Notice the quiet rhythm, inhaling and exhaling, expanding and releasing, filling and letting go, the breath moving in and out. Once you feel relaxed and aware of your witness consciousness, choose any of the following phrases and repeat the words in your mind or aloud. Repeat them without judgment or expectation of any particular outcome or result. Notice what feelings arise or any sensations that might occur in the body. What thoughts may arise in response to the words, without judging the thoughts that may come, simply noticing.

- My thoughts and senses create my reality.
- I exist only in the now.
- I am not this body.
- I am not who I think I am.
- I am infinite.
- All is One.
- I am One.
- Nothing can be lost.

- I am never lost.
- I am never born and can never die.
- Death is birth.
- Birth is death.
- I am peace.
- Nothing is separate.
- I am nowhere.
- I am everywhere.
- Truth is One.
- I can rest in peace.
- I AM.
- *Om Tat Sat* (All That is True).

Chapter 3

Bhakti Yoga

The Path of Devotion

The path of Bhakti yoga is the path of devotion. Sometimes referred to as the path of the heart, it finds its name in the root of the Sanskrit verb *bhaj*, meaning "to share in" as well as "belonging to." Bhakti practitioners focus on devotional love and, through this, eventually come to see the Divine Oneness in everything, in everyone, and to live fully in a state of consciousness soaked in the continuous pure love of God, which is, in the view of the Bhakti tradition, the natural state of the soul.

In classical teachings, the heart of the Bhakti path is the focus of one's love and devotion toward a particular deity with the goal of forming a deeper and more personal relationship with the Divine. Through purity of devotion and an intimately tended personal relationship with the Divine, the devotee's eternal connection to and with pure Divine Love is awakened and realized. Renowned yogini activist Shiva Rea writes in her beautiful book, *Tending the Heart Fire* (2014), "Central to Bhakti is an emphasis on a mystic and loving experience with the Source, a relationship that is often seen as beloved-lover, friend-friend, parent-child, or God-servant" (p.47).

This tradition for millions of people is illuminated in *The Bhagavad Gita*, one of the sacred texts central to the Hindu religion. Often affectionately referred to as *The Gita*, the lyrical 700-verse text describes the relationship between Lord Krishna and the warrior Arjuna in his search for Oneness, and serves as a guide for cultivating the ultimate relationship with the Divine. This text holds the first known reference to *Bhaktimarga*, the path (*marga*) of devotional love, which awakens the presence of Divine Love in our hearts and through which we realize our own true nature of love as well as our eternal connection with the Source.

Love is one, paths are many

The passion and fervor of the Bhakti path of love and devotion is seen in other traditions as well, crossing boundaries through nearly all religions and paths of the world including Hinduism, Christianity, Buddhism, Sufism, Judaism, Islam, as well as tribal and pagan religions. The ecstatic and soulful poems of thirteenth-century Sufi mystic Jalal ad Din Rumi's heartfelt worship of and longing for the Divine continue to move readers more than 700 years after his death. The writings of Saint Teresa of Avila, sixteenth-century Carmelite nun and Spanish Christian mystic, whose deep and avid seeking for her Divine Beloved evokes the mystery and ecstasy of the path of love and longing within all who read her words. The ninenteenth-century Indian mystic and teacher Ramakrishna Paramahansa spoke and wrote of his devout love for and worship of many forms of the One. His objects of devotion included the fierce Hindu goddess Kali, Islam's Allah, as well as Jesus Christ and His mother Mary, demonstrating how the multifaceted, devotional love and worship of the Divine can take many forms and represent many paths.

Christianity is nearly synonymous with the path of love. The focal point of the New Testament, and the crux of all the teachings of Jesus, rests on the ultimate understanding that love of all humanity is the same as the love of God. Jesus said we are to "love the Lord thy God with all thy heart," and to "love thy neighbor as thyself."

The Christian focus on God as Love is an extension of the Judaic tradition in which a primary focus of the religion is the importance of learning to "love the Lord your God with all your heart, and with all your soul and with all your might," as directed in Deuteronomy 6:5. King Solomon's *Song of Songs* is one of the most beautifully written parables of love in existence and is an exquisite example of the Bhakti tradition of describing the relationship of Divine Lover to Devoted Beloved. Using the language of love, the *Song of*

Songs shows us the Divine fire of Love in its all-consuming bliss and delight, as well the ache of separation and desperate longing for unification.

In all the great spiritual paths and religious traditions, love and the power therein is shown over and over to be the primary and abiding force. In *A Sufi Message of Spiritual Liberty*, twentieth-century Sufi teacher Hazrat Inayat Khan interpreted the sacred phrase *Ishq Allah Ma'bud Allah* to mean "God is Love, Lover and Beloved" and taught his students the importance of recognizing God as Love. The Earth-based pagan religion Wicca teaches that "Love is the Law." Love is stronger than death. Love conquers all, and as John, Paul, George and Ringo know and have sung to all of our hearts, "All you need is love."

Bhakti is the yoga way of love and recognizes that love is the primary unfolding and upholding force of the universe, regardless of religion or tradition. The heart of God in all forms can ultimately be understood, known, experienced and seen as the unending fountain from which all blessings and all of creation continually flows. Love sustains and maintains the universe and all that exists within it. Bhakti is the path to immersion and Oneness with and within that love. God is love. Love is God. There is no difference.

The model of the Bhakti relationship to the deity is based on the human to human relationships with which we are familiar: beloved to lover, parent to child, friend to friend, sibling to sibling, student to teacher. Through and within these relationships each of us can find the opportunity to experience deep, pure and true love. The bhakta's relationship to the Divine is based on models of relationships that are human because these types are what we are familiar with. We are limited in these physical forms and cannot easily know or understand the fullness of God in all of God's forms so we must take the roads we know and the roads travel both ways. God is Love and Love is God.

I bow to the Divine in you

Through deep relationship to and with God we can learn better how to love our fellow human beings. Through human-to-human relationships we can also learn how to better love God. Sixteenth-century mystical saint Teresa of Avila wrote in her work *Interior Castle* (2007), "Think of a bright light pouring into a room from two large windows; it enters from different places, but becomes one light" (p.69). Through pure-hearted devotion toward our beloved human others, in whom we can ultimately see and recognize the Divine, the path and ultimate goal of Oneness with the Divine may also be reached.

Most people who have taken a yoga class have seen and most likely engaged in the practice of taking anjali mudra (see Figure 2.1), bowing the head, and saying "*Namaste*" to the teacher, to the other students and to ourselves. The word, and gesture, is a common greeting throughout India. *Nama* means "to bow," *as* is "me," *te* is "you." I bow to you. The bowing and the greeting is in acknowledgement of the Divine within. The Divine in me bows to the Divine in you. I see and honor the love, the light, the beauty, the depth, the fullness, the bounty and the fire of creation that is within you because it is also in me. My soul recognizes your soul. Each of us is an extension of the Divine Source. This common daily practice that can seem trivial, even rote, recognizes that each of us is part of God; that we ourselves are part of the Divine. This is a truly profound act. I see, acknowledge, and bow to the Divine, which makes Its home in your heart and in mine. I bow to you as God. *Namaste.*

When we acknowledge and understand that each of the humans we love and with whom we are in a relationship is an extension of the Divine, as are we ourselves, it makes sense that we can cultivate love and devotion to God, through devotion to our beloveds, both alive and dead. Through that pure love and devotion, Divine love can be shared and awakened. Through Divine love, all love can be freely given and shared. If we understand fully who we truly are, there is no love that is not Divine. Love goes both ways. There is nothing that Love does not serve and nothing that cannot serve Love because Love is the ultimate Law of the Universe and the essence of every form of the Divine. Through devotion and love to others we love and express devotion to the Divine. As Jesus said in Matthew 25:40, "Verily I say unto you, inasmuch as ye have done it unto one of the least of these my brethren, ye have done it unto me."

The spiritual crisis of grief

Through the practice of Jnana yoga, as understood in the second chapter, we can learn that we are not who we think we are. By the light of the Truth testing of Jnana, we can realize and know that our true and unchanging Self is the Divine within. To love our Selves is to love God and to love God is to love our Selves. We are told in commandments, and even more truly by our own hearts, to love all the world as our own True Self, as we love God. We cannot truly do otherwise because the Source is in us and we are in It. We cannot be separate. We are One.

This can be incredibly difficult to know, to remember, to believe or even to contemplate when we are in the midst of deep grief. For some, it can feel impossible. Grief is a spiritual crisis. Questioning God and questioning faith are very normal parts of grief for many bereaved people. The opposite can also occur, as the bereaved may experience the urge to turn toward faith and become immersed in religious practices. Either of these tendencies can be addressed with Bhakti yoga practices. I have also known atheists and agnostics who in the longing for expression of their grief and longing have found a place of spiritual succor through honoring their beloved dead through Bhakti practices.

The spiritual experience of grief can be a crisis as well as an awakening. Because yoga teaches how to hold two opposing thoughts at once, we don't have to choose one or the other, crisis or awakening. Both of these can be a catalyst for change and transformation. Grief is surely a transformative place where we are stripped of our ideas of who we thought we were, how we thought things were, how we thought life was "supposed to be." There is no escaping the space of confrontation with what is. And what is, is that which we never wanted to experience. We never even thought of it as a possibility.

The emergence of new dimensions of consciousness often results from tragic loss. Traumatic grief can bring the griever to a place of stripped down nakedness of self, where ego and identities are destroyed. The bereaved and bereft know this state intimately. Complete vulnerability, emptiness filled with a pain so deep, so pervasive and profound that all else falls away, unimportant, unreal. That feeling can bring with it sacred glimpses into the All. Because we are so wounded, wholly immersed in deep longing for our beloveds, for the way things were, for a reality that we wish desperately to return to, we often cannot fully see, appreciate or embrace the solace that can come from this space of emptiness.

There is deep honesty and authenticity in embracing fully whatever feeling state we are experiencing. It bothers me that, so often, spiritual and self-help books seem to present the opportunity for spiritual growth in opposition to the experience of feeling contracted, closed, even impenetrable in our sorrow. The message is often that those visited by tragedy and grief either resist or they yield. Rarely do the books tell us that we can do both. We can resist it with everything that is in us and we can also yield. We can even do both at the same time.

The dark night of the soul

Imprisoned following attempts to reform the church, sixteenth-century Spanish mystic St. John of the Cross wrote of the spiritual crisis he coined the "dark night of the soul." He wrote:

> The deep suffering of the soul in the night…comes not so much from the aridity she must endure but from this growing suspicion that she has lost her way. She thinks that spiritual blessing is over and that God has abandoned her. She finds neither support nor delight in holy things. Growing weary she struggles in vain to practice the tricks that used to yield results, applying her faculties to some object of meditation in hopes of finding satisfaction. (2002, p.67)

When we are wandering the depths of the dark night, it can be nearly impossible to imagine, much less see, that growth might be happening. The notion that darkness and dark places necessarily must be bad is inherently wrong. The Bible says that, in the beginning, darkness was upon the face of the waters, and then there was light. It says too that the light was good, but it does not say that the dark was bad. The darkness came before the light. Perhaps the light first needed the dark in order to shine forth.

Darkness nurtures and supports innumerable types of growth and life. Seeds must be planted in the deep soil of the Earth and allowed to germinate in the dark. Tiny pods swell, expand and eventually burst forth tiny tendrils of growth under cover of dark. In the dark of night, countless nocturnal creatures thrive: bats, owls, cats of all kinds—domestic, jungle and mountain—lemurs, opossum, deer, rabbits, scorpions, fireflies and more. A plethora of plants bloom and grow only in absence of light. You will never see the glory of a night-blooming jasmine or the ethereal beauty of the pale moonflower flourish in the harsh light of day.

The caterpillar conducts its total transformation enveloped in the dark sheath of its chrysalis. In swaddled darkness, its body dissolves completely, becoming unrecognizable goo. Within the goo are special cells called imago cells which contain the specific instructions for transforming the goo into a winged creature of air and sun. To become a butterfly, the caterpillar is literally liquefied and then, by a force that unfolds only in darkness, is reconfigured into a creature that looks and acts totally differently from the one that went into the darkness. Caterpillars experience complete dissolution and reconfiguration into something wholly new and different. It's not very glamorous and is surely painful. Ask the caterpillar. If you are a person who has experienced deep grief, this process should sound at least somewhat familiar.

The process of dissolution in transformation is something that we have very little control over. When we feel that we must control it, manage it, do it better, have a specific outcome or do it the way other people want us to do it, we (and they) can be sorely disappointed. Transformation, and the ultimate resultant growth, is only postponed when we try to make it something it is not. But this is okay too. As much as we might want a schedule, or as much as others may want us to have one, a schedule for grieving, or for transformation and potential resultant growth, does not exist.

It is a rare individual who in the face of deep grief has not felt lost, closed or unable to be helped. We may go in and out of states of self-pity, resentment, feeling aggrieved and unfairly treated by the universe, to states of deep gratitude for having had such a love, for each breath we take, for each tiny blade of grass. This process of back and forth is part of the dissolution and transformation. I don't believe we must be *either* full of the peace that passes understanding *or* a victim of grief wallowing in self-pity. I don't think it must be an either/or option. It can be both/and.

Several years passed following my son Theo's death before I could read or hear anything remotely spiritually tinged without an undercurrent of hostility and bitterness. Sometimes, the feeling was outright anger and unequivocal rejection of what was being shared. Beneath the anger was fear, pain and a sense of unworthiness, the feeling that I was unable to be helped by anyone, that I was doing it all wrong. Rarely did I read or hear that it was okay to feel whatever I was feeling. Instead the message seemed to be if I was not opening with gratitude and turning toward the incredible shimmering beauty that is inherent in the time-limited opportunity that is life, then I was somehow deficient. I knew of course, that much of this was my projection, my perception, my limited internal experience. But it was incredibly visceral and real. My whole body, mind, heart and spirit cried out, railing against what was happening. Here was the fire of grief and pain and shock and intense longing, yearning, for my child. This was unfair! Unfair! And yes, it was.

I also had times of incredible peace and lightness of being, like the moment in my bathtub when I felt immersed not merely in a tub of warm water and salty tears, but in the timeless ocean of the All. Chanting the opening verse of the *Isha Upanishad*, a deep and full understanding of the ancient vibrations of *purnamidah* came into my being, the veil of grief lifted, if only for a moment. I will never forget that experience. That moment sustained me and continues to sustain me in times of doubt and spiritual struggle. Interestingly, many early moments of peace I remember occurred in and near water.

Being in or around water seems always to remind me that even in my anguish, there is always the love. Love is always there. It is always the love that softens the anger and allows the pain to be endured. Love is naturally present and never dissipates even with the presence of the deepest pain. Swami Prabhavananda wrote in his translation and commentary on the

Hindu saint *Narada's Way of Divine Love*, that the path of Bhakti "is the most natural and easy path. For everyone has love in his heart, only this love has to be directed toward God." I believe directing love toward our beloveds is one and the same as directing love toward God in a different form.

All forms of water flow eventually, inevitably into the all-embracing body of the ocean. Perhaps the form is a trickling stream, a majestic waterfall, an undulating pool, a rain shower, an angry thundering storm, a frozen glacier, a breaking wave, a soft mist. The ocean eventually embraces all forms of water. It does not forget or cast aside the smallest of waves, even when the wave does not know or remember that it is part of the ocean, the ocean receives the wave into itself, over and over. Love takes different forms in different people. We are each a droplet of water from the Divine Sea of Love. The ocean does not see the wave as separate from itself, even if the wave sees itself as separate from the ocean.

Meditation

Breathing in, I am the wave; breathing out, I am the ocean

This meditation can be done anywhere, any time. It can remind us of our essential connectedness to each other and to Spirit.

Find a comfortable spot. Sit comfortably with your spine straight but not stiff. Close the eyes and begin to notice the flow of your breath as it moves into the body, the expansion of the abdomen, the ribcage, the chest, the subtle movements perhaps of the shoulders, the collarbones. Notice as the exhalation leaves the body, softly, the air warmed by the temperature of the body, the change in the belly, the ribs, the chest. Follow the breath as it comes in and as it goes out. Slightly deepen the breath, allowing the belly and the low ribs and the back to expand further with each inhalation. Allow the inhale and the exhale to be of equal length. Continue to gently allow the inhale to become even deeper, the belly, the ribs, the back of the body, the chest expanding gently. Pausing slightly at the crest of the inhalation, let the exhalation gently release the breath, chest, ribs and belly moving down and in. Continue to allow the inhalation and exhalation to be of equal length.

As you inhale this slow, easy deep breath, imagine, as if in slow motion, a gentle wave, rising, building and swelling. See the gentle, cool light of a full moon caressing the edges of the water, reflected in the curve of the wave as it rises. As it crests, allow the wave to pause in a moment of stillness. As the wave is released back toward the sea, it gently unfurls into its source, disappearing into the depths. There is another pause and the wave begins to rise again.

Let the breath move in and out of the body using no force, as if it flows in and out on its own with no struggle. The breath moves continuously, in and out, like the tide pulled eternally by the forces of Earth and Moon. Breathing in, imagine yourself as the wave, rising, reflecting the light of the soft glow of the moon, cresting, pausing, and then sinking once again.

Inhaling, rising.

Exhaling, sinking.

Imagine the fullness of the ocean taking you, as this wave, lovingly back into itself.

Breathing in…think, *"I am the wave."*

Breathing out…think, *"I am the ocean."*

Continue as long as you wish. When you are ready to stop the meditation, gently open the eyes.

Yoga in all its paths shows us again and again that there is an infinite well of love which is Divine and part of everything and everyone, whether we feel connected to it or not. There is no judgment or fault or punishment if we don't recognize our connectedness or the presence of the Divine in all things and in all people. The teachings of yoga hold that when we are ready to realize the connection, we will.

In channeling and expressing our deep love for those who have died, we can begin to facilitate the kind of connection to Spirit that the path of Bhakti invariably leads us toward. Bhakti is not necessarily a path for everyone but, as Swami Prabhavanada tells us, it is thought to be the easiest. Bhakti is the state of being consumed by devotion and pure Divine Love. There are many ways to get there. Truth is One, Paths are Many.

Creating shrines and altars

Archeologists have found evidence of shrines and altars, sacred creations, in virtually all places where humans have lived. Traditionally, shrines are memorials, or monuments, to the dead. People have created shrines for thousands of years and across all cultures. Some well-known shrines include the Taj Mahal and the Egyptian pyramids. Memorials such as the Martin Luther King Memorial, the Vietnam Veterans' Memorial, the Mount Rushmore carvings, and the Lincoln Memorial are examples of secular shrines that honor the memories of our respected and revered dead.

People create shrines in public spaces and communities as well as in homes and in places of worship. Think of those we can see along the sides of roads and highways where someone died in a car crash. These spaces are sacred to the family and those who loved that person. Often the place where a person died is more important than a burial space. Public and community shrines may be created and added to spontaneously at sites of tragedies, such as those created by students, faculty and families at Columbine or Virginia Tech after the tragic shootings that took place in those schools, or in neighborhoods where tragedies have taken place. Shrines may be created outside homes or at the burial sites of well-loved public figures or artists who have died such as those created in honor of John Lennon, Princess Diana, Jim Morrison and Edgar Allan Poe. Shrines certainly serve as places for solitude and reflection but can also be whimsical and celebratory like the brightly colored Day of the Dead shrines in Mexico's annual festivities which celebrate and honor the lives of loved ones with parades, games, picnics and family gatherings.

An altar is generally considered a specific, sacred space used for worship, prayer, offerings or other religious and spiritual purposes. In religious traditions, the altar is usually the centerpiece of the worship space, such as in a church, synagogue, temple or mosque. Many people create home altars as a personal sacred space for prayer, reflection or meditation. Home altars can help focus our minds on our chosen spiritual path and serve as daily reminders of a spiritual focus or our connection to Spirit.

Altars and shrines are external representations of interior mysteries. They are ways of showing in tangible form what is happening in our hearts and spirits. Creating shrines and altars gives us opportunity to remember, reflect and honor those we love who have died as well as transform pain through the creative act (Figure 3.1).

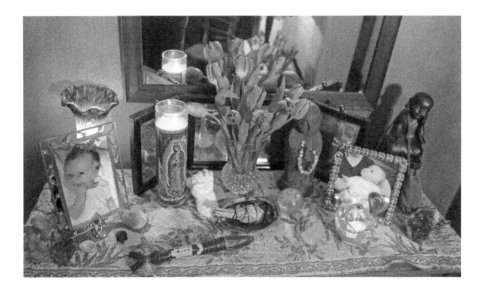

Figure 3.1 Home altar.

Often, the words altar and shrine are used interchangeably. You can use whichever term you prefer or you may wish to think of a personally created altar or shrine as a memorial, memory box, memory space, meditation place, honoring space or simply a special place. It can be whatever you choose. The creation is a sacred, expressive act of love, a practice of the Bhakti path. The finished piece ultimately helps us to center our feelings of devotion and love toward the focal points of the shrine. It helps us to enter into sacred space. Each time you light a candle or sit quietly focusing on the pictures or other sacred objects that are part of your creation, you are performing a Bhakti practice.

Portable shrines (Figure 3.2) can be carried with you wherever you go. These might be as small as a matchbook that can fit in your pocket or something a bit larger, like the size of a book, for instance, that might be slipped into a purse or briefcase. A smaller, take-along shrine allows you to maintain connection with your loved one, or to have the means to create sacred space for remembering or engaging in a personal ritual any time or place you need or want to do so. You might prefer to create a semi-permanent shrine or altar whose elements can be taken apart and used in other places or spaces. Or you may wish to create a more permanent shrine or altar space that will be a focal point of a room or outdoor space. The choices are yours.

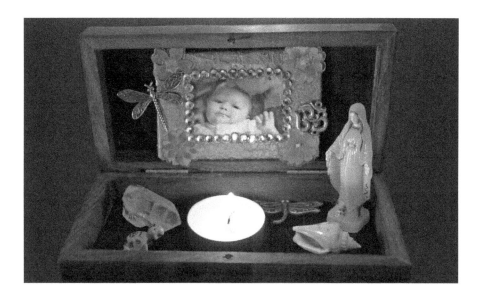

Figure 3.2 Travel altar.

Experiential practice
Creating your shrine

There are no rules or guidelines for creating shrines. The beauty of creating a shrine is that the ideas and materials are seemingly endless and the process, like grieving, is completely individual. Before you plan the look of your shrine, you may want to spend some time thinking about your loved one, without thoughts or preconceived ideas of what you think your shrine will or should look like.

Here are some suggestions that may help the process:

- Make a list of words that come to mind when you think of your loved one.
- Make a list of objects or things that you associate with your loved one.
- Write down any words of wisdom, favorite expressions, funny or loving things your beloved may have said.
- Write down nicknames or pet names you might have used for each other and write down any associations those words may bring up.
- Write down his or her favorite colors, flowers, foods, hobbies, talents, etc.
- Research and find images that correspond to some of the things you have listed. You may find lots of interesting images on the internet that you can print and cut out for use in your creation. The images you encounter may spark other thoughts or ideas that you may wish to incorporate in your memorial shrine.

To create a permanent shrine

I always suggest that a container be decided on first before proceeding. The container may help guide the process or selection of items used in creating your shrine. If you know you want to build a more permanent shrine, even if it is a small one, be on the lookout for containers or objects that speak to you, or seem to call out to be repurposed into your very own sacred space.

Some suggestions for containers which can be repurposed as shrines:

- Altoid tins (or other candy or gum tins)
- sliding matchboxes
- jewelry boxes
- gift boxes
- shoe boxes
- deep frames or shadow boxes
- drawers
- books (you can make a book into a box by cutting a rectangular shape into the pages and then gluing the pages together to create a container inside the book)
- small pieces of furniture like stools, small cabinets, side tables or plant stands.

Gather together your basic supplies:

- scissors
- glue (I prefer acrylic gel medium)
- paints (acrylic craft paints are inexpensive and work very well for this purpose)
- decorative and/or colored papers
- photographs, personal objects or other items related to your loved one
- anything else that you wish to add to your creation, such as ribbons, wires, sticks, dried flowers, string, yarn, decorative paper, wrapping paper, rhinestones, shells, small mirrors, glitter, charms or beads.

Then, begin your process.

- Prepare your surface by painting or covering the outside and then the inside of your container, allow it to dry completely. Using gesso to prepare the surface can be helpful before adding color.
- Add background papers or images on the prepared surface if you wish.

- Place the photo(s) of your loved one where you think it should go.

- Add embellishments, representations of the Divine, other meaningful objects and other elements as desired inside and out including beads, glass pieces, pebbles, shells, words, charms, etc., until you feel you have completed your shrine.

To create a semi-permanent shrine or altar space

You may choose to forgo the paints, glues and embellishments. To create a semi-permanent shrine, decide on your location or designate a particular space, such as a table top or a special shelf. You may want to visit thrift and antique shops to find the perfect small table or shelf that will serve as the base for your home altar/shrine. Once you've found your base, begin the assembling of your sacred space.

Gather together meaningful items that will help you focus on your love as well as your intent to memorialize, remember and honor. You may wish to cover your altar with a special cloth or decorative mat. Next, you may want to place a picture of your beloved in a special frame as the centerpiece of your shrine. Add to this basic memorial anything you wish. Some suggestions might include:

- personal objects that remind you of, or are connected to, your beloved (these might include jewelry, letters or cards he or she gave you, awards, trophies, hats and other items of clothing, favorite books, something he or she used on a regular basis such as sewing scissors, razor, comb or brush)

- photos or other representations of a chosen deity; these may be statues, photos, icons

- natural objects such as flowers, fruits, rocks, crystals, shells, sticks or branches from your back yard, pinecones, leaves, abandoned birds' nests, etc.

- candles, incense

- chimes or bells.

You may add to or change the objects on your shrine as often as you wish. You can use your shrine or altar space simply as a reminder of your loved one or as an active part of creating and conducting personal grief rituals and Bhakti devotional practices.

Temporary nature shrines

You may also choose to create a completely temporary shrine in nature— in the woods, a park or in your own back yard. Choose a space outdoors, a flat rock, an appealing open space on the ground, a nook of a tree, any outdoor space you find pleasing and where you are not disturbing existing animal homes or harming any natural life. Place stones, shells, flowers or other natural objects in pleasing arrangements in your chosen space. You may want to create a cairn with stacked stones, or a medicine wheel with pebbles, sticks and seashells (see Figure 3.3). You may choose to leave bird seed, nuts or bits of fruit as offerings to nature. After you construct your outdoor sacred space, sit for as long as you wish to pray, chant, meditate or speak to your beloved. You can choose to leave the sacred configuration of natural items as they are or disassemble the space when you leave.

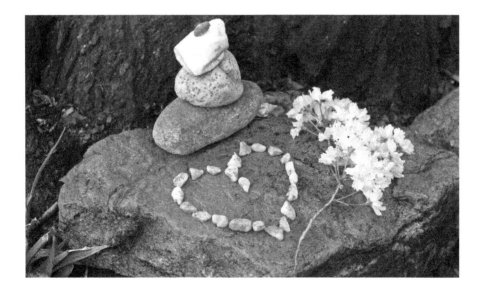

Figure 3.3 Stone cairn.

Grief as love's expression:
Transformation in sacred spaces

Deep grief exists because of deep love. If we never loved, we would never grieve. How many would relinquish love to be free of grief? I would wager not many. The Bhakti path teaches that through love, all emotions, from joy to pain, anger to gratitude, are acknowledged, accepted, directed and, ultimately, facilitate movement toward realization of our Oneness with the Source which is Love.

In Bhakti practice, all feelings, emotions and experiences in grief, as in all emotions, are welcome. The bhakta's complete absorption in the beloved, her forgetting of ego and self, her surrender to powerlessness in the face of intense love and the fire of devotion are entirely understandable to the profoundly bereaved whose experience of intense emotion is part of daily existence in grief. The place of deep love and longing for our beloved dead is sacred space. It is in that sacred space that transformation occurs.

Grief and love are equally transformative. Emergent realties about who we are, who we thought we once were, and the impact of grief on our lives are inescapable. Like the caterpillar, we are dissolved. Like it or not, we are changed. Life will never be the same again. We may have no idea what is going on, or what may happen next; we are in the midst of metamorphosis. Through trust in Love, the True Self can be allowed to unfold like new wings. In his teachings on *Bhakti Yoga: The Yoga of Love and Devotion* (2013), Swami Vivekananda wrote that "with perfect love, true knowledge is bound to come even unsought, and that from perfect knowledge true love is inseparable"(p.7).

Embracing grief as love's expression opens the way for transformation. Pain as love can be endured and even willingly approached. Pain melting into love can soothe, ease and gently open the closed, guarded and wounded spaces within. With love, the heart expands to allow grief a sacred space.

The transformation of pain includes not only seeing grief as love, but finding within us the strength to approach it, to sit with it, to examine it, to be immersed in it; even if we feel afraid, sick, pained or in a thousand other ways averse to the experience. In all relationships, love grows, love evolves, love changes. Grief also changes shape, form and intensity as do our individual experiences, expressions, and our relationships to and with it.

This next experiential meditation asks that you visualize a concrete image of your grief. By engaging with images of our grief, the phenomenon of grief's mutability, and the changeable nature of our relationship with and to it can be more easily understood. While this exercise can certainly be anxiety-producing, directly approaching grief—or allowing it to approach you—is much more helpful and ultimately less threatening than dealing with grief unnamed, amorphous, continually pushed away. Finding mindful ways to hold, honor and expand your love by turning toward, moving into and creatively engaging with grief is inherent to the practices of Bhakti.

Meditation

Being with your grief

Find a comfortable, safe space where you will remain undisturbed for the duration of this meditation. You may wish to do this exercise in the presence of or with guidance from a trusted friend or therapist.

Begin by sitting comfortably. Let your spine be long but not stiff. Allow your hands to be open and relaxed. Take a few deep, cleansing, centering breaths. Begin to become aware of your body. Mentally scan the body from the soles of your feet to the top of your head, becoming conscious of any places in the body where you may be holding stress or tension. Notice your feet, knees, legs, hips, belly, chest, back, hands, arms, shoulders, neck, face and head. Notice any twinges, any pain, any stiffness or unease. Notice discomfort or comfort. Notice your heartbeat—is it fast or slow? Notice the breath as it moves in and out of the body. Notice and label, if you can, any emotions you may be experiencing right now.

As you inhale, imagine sending your breath, and the energizing life-giving force that it carries, into any spaces where you may be feeling discomfort or tension. Imagine your muscles growing softer and more relaxed while your bones hold you steady and firm. Begin to notice the temperature of the air on your skin. Notice the feel of the floor beneath your feet, the pressure of the chair or cushion holding your weight. Know that you are held and that you are safe. Right here and right now. Continue to be aware of your breath as it moves in and out of the body.

When you are ready, begin to visualize a safe space. You might imagine yourself in a comforting space where you spent time with your beloved, in a favorite room from your past or present, or in a place of nature. This may be special place you have visited before and have used previously as a mental, emotional, or spiritual refuge. Or, it may be a brand new place, a wholly imagined space all your own. Whatever and wherever it is, it is your space. It is safe. Allow yourself to be present in that special, safe space. See yourself sitting peacefully and with ease in that space. Imagine the surroundings; see the colors, the objects and shapes that surround you. Notice details such as textures, smells and sounds. Perhaps you hear the rustle of leaves, or maybe there is music or birdsong nearby. Look around and feel completely comfortable, safe and secure in this space.

When you feel ready, allow your grief to take form. Know that, as grief takes form, you continue to remain safe. From your place of safety, look upon your grief. Notice what your grief looks like. What form does it take? How close or how far away is your grief? Know that you are in charge of the distance between you and your grief in this moment. Your grief is yours alone. It is completely unique to you. It may take the form of a person, a shape, an object or an elemental representation. It may appear as something that exists in nature or solely in your imagination. Whatever form your grief takes is the form that it is supposed to be in this moment, at this time. Know that you continue to remain safe and supported.

Knowing that you are safe, allow your grief in its form to approach you. Allow it to come as slowly as you wish. You are in control of its approach. You control the amount of space between you and your grief. Notice whether you can get a closer look. What details do you notice about your grief? How does it move? Are there sounds? Is there motion? Notice the size of your grief relative to the surroundings.

In the presence of grief, how do you feel?

Where do you feel the sensations in your body?

When you are ready, begin a dialogue with grief. Ask your grief, "What is your name?" Ask it, "Why are you named that?"

What does your grief have to tell you?

What do you have to say to your grief?

Tell grief if there is something you would like to change about your relationship to it, to him, to her. Tell grief anything else that you would like it to know. Perhaps you might want to tell grief something about you, about your journey, about how you feel with it as a constant companion, about how it feels to you, what emotions you experience because of it, how it feels in your body, about what has happened since grief came to your life. Perhaps there are other things you might want to say.

In this moment you can begin a dialogue with grief that can continue all your life. Say whatever you wish; ask whatever you want to ask. Listen to the answers. You did not choose this grief, but it is now a part of your life. Here it is, ready to be seen, to listen and perhaps, to speak. Whatever occurs in this encounter with your grief is exactly what needs to occur.

When you are ready to leave this particular experience with grief, begin to become aware of your body once more in this present moment. Notice the feel of the floor beneath you, the seat upon which you rest. Become aware of any sounds in the space around you. Come back into this present reality. Take a deep breath and open your eyes.

Write about this experience in your journal; discuss it with a trusted friend or therapist. Know that you can come back to this safe space to continue a dialogue with grief anytime you want or need to.

Paint, draw, collage or otherwise create a portrait of your grief or another kind of representation of your experience in this space with grief.

When grief comes again, as it will, into your everyday life, imagine that the feelings and experiences you will have are visits from the form that your grief took during this meditation. Imagine the continuation of the dialogue that began here. Notice how your reaction and your relationship to and with grief may change over time. This exercise can be a lifelong tool to help you be with the changing nature of grief as it is, time after time.

This meditation is a gratefully adapted version of an exercise from Dr. Joanne Cacciatore's workbook *Selah: An Invitation Toward Fully Inhabited Grief* (2013).

Turning love inward

We can learn to be present with grief and to know that while grief would not exist if not for love, grief can never overpower the love. We can learn to have a relationship to and with grief, while continuing to grow and express love. We can do this through actively and mindfully finding expression of love through devotion, ritual, remembrance and, as the Karma chapter addresses, through turning love outward, toward others. We can also find love's expression through love of self, self-care, self-compassion and through mindful awareness of where we are individually in our grief and how we relate to grief at various moments in time.

We can learn and know that even though we may feel the pain of grief deeply, immensely, though we may fear or dread the pain, it will not kill us. If we do not acknowledge it, we can become more undone than if we turn toward it and allow it expression. Shakespeare entreated us to "Give sorrow words; the grief that does not speak knits up the o'erwrought heart and bids it break." Unexpressed grief can be poison. Turning toward and expressing grief allows transmutation. Expression of our love allows us to begin to see love elsewhere. We can open to compassion for others. We can begin to allow grief to make space for joy.

Yoga is a great teacher of how to hold two opposing thoughts. Rumi told us, "The grief you cry out from draws you toward union" (p.78). Grief and joy can reside alongside each other. Love makes possible the opening and growth of those new spaces. It takes practice to do this, and yoga is a continual practice. Everything is a practice and nothing is perfect, except your True Self, which is and has always been perfect. The way of yoga provides practice for us to come to this realization of our divine perfection and all that entails, which when realized, allows us to be free from pain. When you are immersed in a never-ending ocean of love, you don't have to let go of the pain. The pain will eventually let go of you.

Metta meditation

Loving the self

Metta Meditation is a Buddhist practice which helps us move into a state of self-love and compassion, and then further into love and compassion toward others. I am a firm believer that we cannot give away what we don't have. It will not be possible to give or practice genuine love and compassion toward others if we cannot give it first to ourselves.

To practice, find a comfortable place to sit. Take a few deep, cleansing breaths. Begin to center and bring yourself into the present moment. Do this by beginning to notice the space around you. Close your eyes if that feels comfortable. If not, find a spot on the floor a few feet in front of you and allow your gaze to soften. This is always an option when meditating. As you sit, begin to notice the temperature of the air on your skin. Notice any sounds you may hear outside the room; notice any sounds you may hear inside your own space. Notice the feel of the floor beneath your feet. Notice the pressure of the chair or the floor under your sitting bones and your legs. Notice the weight of your body as it is supported. Expand your awareness by beginning to notice sensations throughout your body. Scan the body from the bottoms of your feet to the top of your head, moving slowly through each body part, noticing any places of tension or stress.

When you reach the top of your head, move the awareness back down, checking the face, the neck, the shoulders, arms, hands, back, chest, belly, hips, legs, knees, calves, ankles and feet for tension and stress. Simply notice what is. If you wish, shift or change any space that feels discomfort until you feel more at ease.

Begin to notice and follow the flow of your breath as it moves in and out of your body, inhaling and exhaling. As you inhale, notice the temperature and the feel of the air as it flows through your nasal passages, down your throat and trachea, to your lungs. Notice the different sensations of the belly, the ribs and the chest as they expand. As you exhale, notice the temperature of the air, any movement of the air through the nostrils. Notice the feeling of your lungs filling and emptying of air as the breath comes in and leaves your body. Simply notice these things and any other sensations that occur as you continue to breathe, easily and naturally, in and out.

Bring your awareness to the spaces between inhalation and exhalation. As you become aware of that space between breaths, bring your awareness then to your heart center. In the space between breaths, we can feel, sense and hear the beat of our hearts. If you place your fingers on the carotid artery, just below your jawbone, you can begin to feel the sonic vibration, the internal sound waves of your heartbeat. As you hold your fingers on the pulse, begin to notice the vibration of the beat of your heart within the ears.

Shift your awareness fully to the heart space, where the vibrations of love and the fullness of all our feelings emanate. If you wish, you can visualize a sphere of green or pink light radiating from your heart center. You may wish to cross your hands over the center of your chest in *svastika* mudra (Figure 3.4), meaning cross. This mudra creates the same energy as anjali mudra with a reverent, intimate and loving quality directed inwardly, toward the self. You may wish to visualize the green or pink light at your heart center growing with each beat of your heart until it encompasses you fully in a protective, loving sphere. This is the energy of your own heart.

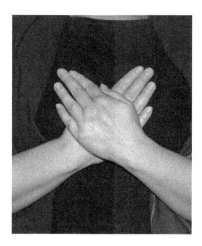

Figure 3.4 Svastika mudra.

Once you feel your heart energy and establish space within your sphere of light, begin to repeat, mentally or aloud, these phrases of loving-kindness:

May I be peaceful and at ease.

May I be well in body, mind and heart.

May I accept myself completely, just as I am in this moment.

May I be held perpetually in loving-kindness.

In your mind's eye, imagine that you can float outside your own body and see yourself sitting encompassed within that sphere of light. Notice from what perspective you are seeing the image of yourself. Hold this image.

In this second repetition of the phrases of loving-kindness, imagine directing the phrases as waves of energy toward the image of your own precious self sitting encompassed within the sphere of light and love which emanates from your own heart center.

May I be peaceful and at ease.

May I be well in body, mind and heart.

May I accept myself completely, just as I am in this moment.

May I be held perpetually in loving-kindness.

If feelings of love, warmth, friendliness or peacefulness arise in the body, allow yourself to connect to them. Sink into your own genuine intention for these sincerely expressed wishes for blessings of kindness, peace and love toward yourself. If it is helpful, imagine your beloved dead, as well as other spirit guides and ancestors, joining with you to send loving-kindness toward your own dearest self. Imagine these wishes coming to you from your beloved out of the infinite space of peace and love. Imagine them standing near you, just behind you or at your shoulder. Know that they send these loving wishes toward you as well.

Continue to repeat the phrases of loving-kindness toward yourself until you feel a natural pause in your repetitions. When this occurs, bring to mind an image of a friend, a family member or other person in your life who has deeply cared for you. Repeat the phrases of loving-kindness, directing them now toward that person. You may choose to expand your sphere of heart light to include the person you are thinking of. Imagine that person sitting or standing in the space with you. Continue to repeat the phrases in this way:

May you be peaceful and at ease.

May you be well in body, mind and heart.

May you accept yourself completely, just as you are in this moment.

May you be held perpetually in loving-kindness.

Continue until you feel a natural pause and then bring to mind other friends, family members, neighbors, animal companions, co-workers, acquaintances, anyone you who comes to mind. Continue to repeat the phrases, directing them toward those loved ones.

May you be peaceful and at ease.

May you be well in body, mind and heart.

May you accept yourself completely, just as you are in this moment.

May you be held perpetually in loving-kindness.

Continue to expand the sphere of your heart light and direct loving-kindness toward and including all these loved ones. If feelings of love, warmth, friendliness, peacefulness arise, allow yourself to connect to those feelings. Allow these feelings to energize, fill and direct the phrases of loving-kindness as you repeat them.

At another pause, begin to expand the energy and quality of your meditation to include the entire world, the entire universe. This may sound extreme, but if we think about it, it is not. Energy directed from our minds and hearts is powerful. Like other kinds of waves—radio, sound, light—the energy waves created by our thought waves, particularly when purposefully directed, can have great reach and great power. Just as all other forms of energy waves are emitted from a source and travel across galaxies, so do our thought waves. We can encompass all beings in loving-kindness energy.

May all beings everywhere be peaceful and at ease.

May all beings everywhere be well in body, mind and heart.

May all beings everywhere accept themselves completely, just as they are in this moment.

May all beings everywhere be held perpetually in loving-kindness.

At times during loving-kindness, as well as other types of meditation, feelings may arise that are uncomfortable, unwanted, seemingly the opposite of what you are trying to accomplish. This is a sign that our hearts are softening toward the great pain and suffering of not only our own experiences, but that of other beings across our world and the universe. Try to harbor no judgment toward yourself or the practice and allow the feelings to be what they are. If possible, direct the energy of loving-kindness toward those feelings. There may be sadness, anxiety, pain, confusion, judgment, anger, indignance, discontent, uncertainty.

Allow all feelings to be okay. They are feelings. They will shift and change. If you can remain non-judgmental and direct your beam of loving-kindness toward the feelings themselves, you may experience a further melting toward the feelings, seeing their passage into the void. If they are too difficult to tolerate, shift your awareness from the undesirable feelings, thoughts or images to your breath. In and out. You don't have to change anything. Remember that breath moves of its own accord and can help guide you back to yourself. Breathe in. Breathe out.

Complete your meditation by again reminding yourself of the loving-kindness you sent toward yourself earlier. Repeat once more the loving-kindness phrases directed toward yourself. Feel as though the entire universe supports you in your intent to cultivate this love toward yourself.

May I be peaceful and at ease.

May I be well in body, mind and heart.

May I accept myself completely, just as I am in this moment.

May I be held in perpetually loving-kindness.

End with any phrase or word from any tradition that signals the ending of prayer or ritual. Thank you, So Mote it Be, Amen, In the Name of Jesus, Namo Amida Buddha (I Trust in the Buddha of Immeasurable Light), Om Shanti, Shanti, Shanti (Om, Peace, Peace, Peace), or any other ending phrase that you like.

Devotional love

In 1670, French physicist Blaise Pascal wrote in his famous treatise *Pensées*, "There is a God-shaped vacuum in the heart of every person, and it can never be filled by any created thing. It can only be filled by God." Pascal was Christian, but this is not solely a Christian concept. It isn't even a religious concept necessarily. It is a spiritual issue, separate from religion. Religion can certainly support a personal relationship with the Divine, but religion does not guarantee such a thing. True relationship is heart-felt and heart-centered and occurs between the devotee and the Divine. The God-shaped hole, as the concept is often called by theists and philosophers, can be seen as an intrinsic longing for the sacred, the transcendent, the esoteric; a searching for communion and connection to something greater than ourselves.

Many bereaved have told me about private and personal, even secret, practices of praying to their beloveds, sometimes in absence of the ability to pray to God, sometimes when they had never prayed to anyone or anything before, sometimes because it feels more intimate and comforting than praying to a God that perhaps no longer makes sense. Several shared that they had never told anyone else this, thinking they were the only ones who did such a thing. Thinking that others might think they were crazy, that it might be blasphemous. Thinking they were somehow elevating their loved ones to divine status and somehow this was wrong. For me, this only confirms our inner knowledge that our beloved dead are extensions of the Divine. This is a spontaneous Bhakti practice.

It is much easier to recognize the spark of the Divine in those we love deeply than in ourselves. In prayers to their beloved dead, some bereaved ask for intercession, some for strength, and some for help in finding solace. Others confide that they regularly dispatch the spirits of their loved ones outward to impart peace, healing and love. They ask their beloved dead to visit other grieving relatives—grandparents, parents, spouses, siblings, friends—to bring ease, calm, and peace to others who are grieving or who may need help seemingly from beyond this world.

The tendency to turn our prayer lives, meditation, and other contemplative practices toward our beloved dead is a natural and intuitive action. We intuit that our beloveds, being immersed fully in Divine energy, can serve as intercessors, conduits or connections to Grace. We can use our love for them as our means of connection to the All. Even when we cannot feel or recognize the Divine, we can always turn to love, which can help us know that the Divine has never left us. It's not possible.

Bhakti practices are a beautiful way to creatively transform sorrow into the realization of love. There is no lover who does not long to express the depth of his love to his beloved, no parent who does not wish her beloved child to know how deeply she loves and cares for him. Love is one of the easiest and most natural emotions to feel and to express. It is a feeling that nearly all of us have experienced at some point. When that is untrue, it because we have been damaged, made to feel that we are unsafe in expressing or feeling love. To learn to feel and express love once again is a practice that can bring great reward.

Bhakti is about the fire of the heart and its all-consuming love. Because love is universally understood and felt, there are many ways we can cultivate practices of devotion and dedication. The practices of Bhakti love and devotion to our loved ones do not have to be relegated to grief practices. In my yoga teacher training, each branch of yoga was discussed and workshops held with swamis and learned yogis to help us as students better understand each branch. When we were discussing Bhakti yoga, the speaker began telling us how she first realized a living example of Bhakti devotion through seeing love personified in the relationship of June Carter Cash and Johnny Cash. The comparison made much more sense to me later after I reflected on and wrote about how before our son Theo's death, both my husband and I had become bhaktas in pure devotion to our son.

At first look, our dining room appeared to have been transformed into a hospital room. Our beloved child propped on a small mountain of pillows and foam wedges, attached to tubes and feeding machine; his small body surrounded by baskets and drawers full of medical supplies. In the next room, kitchen counter and cabinets overflowed with medicine, syringes, copies of medication and feeding schedules. Looking beyond those things, it was obvious that our home had been transformed into a temple of love and devotion. Every act of care was one of love and devotion to him. All of our lives were transformed. And continue to be transformed. That love does not die.

Journaling exercise

Bhakti devotion in action

When in your life can you recall engaging in actions of pure love and devotion to your loved one, either before or after death? When we do things through our actions, spoken words or created objects, with the intent to communicate pure love and devotion, we are practicing Bhakti in action. During times of sickness, trauma or stress, we all can experience frustration, fear, irritation, anger and anxiety. These are not the times I am asking you to reflect upon. Rather think of a time in your life, either with your loved one who has died, or with someone else whom you love, when your actions and words were purely devoted to that other's ease, peace, comfort and support.

If you can recall times you have done this, you already have practice as a bhakta. What acts can you recall? What was the energy and tone of your action, your motivation, your words and deeds? Write about that time. You may choose to write a short narrative about that moment in time. You can create a poem, as short or as long as you wish. You might simply jot down notes or phrases that recall those memories. You might choose to do an art journal entry, creating in images with photographs, magazine cut-outs, drawing, painting or other forms of mixed media. You are representing a moment in time when your words, thoughts, actions and deeds were fully focused on devotion and love of another. This is a holy and sacred act and, in your rendering of this, allow your writing or other creative action to reflect that sense of the sacred. This is Bhakti practice.

Expanding love: Meditations, mantra and mudra practices to open, soothe and strengthen the heart

The love cultivated through Bhakti practices can be expressed more fully when we are in touch with the energy of our hearts. When our heart energy is fuller and more robust, we are able to better express and expand love. In grief, our heart energy can be depleted and diminished. The metaphor of a broken heart is not merely cliché or so much symbolic language. Our hearts feel and experience the pain of grief and loss physically, emotionally, energetically and spiritually.

Broken Heart Syndrome is a known medical condition in which the heart's pumping function is temporarily disrupted, and sudden chest pain occurs; people report feeling as if they are having a heart attack. Blood tests show no signs of heart damage, no blockage of the arteries and there is ballooning and unusual movement in the left ventricle. The condition usually reverses itself within a week, but occurs following extremely stressful situations. Many cases of this phenomenon occur after experiences of traumatic grief. There is very little that Western medicine can do for this situation. This is because the heart and the energy field surrounding the heart are deeply affected and disturbed by the stress and pain of grief and loss. Our physical bodies respond to energetic and emotional pain.

While we cannot see our energy body in the physical sense, we have all experienced movement of energy in, around and through our bodies. In the Tantra yoga chapter, you will read further about your energetic and subtle bodies, known in yoga as the *koshas*, a Sanskrit word meaning "sheaths." The koshas are concentric layers of our being, conceived of as sheaths or coverings that move from our outermost layer, the physical body, inward to our eternal core. Each of our koshas interacts with and affects the others. Energy flows through and around all of the koshas.

The centers of this flowing energy are known as *chakras*. Chakras, a Sanskrit word meaning "wheel," are often described as whirling vortexes of energy and are located in the second kosha, the body of breath and energy, which is situated next to our physical layer of being. While not visible in the physical body, the main chakras do correspond with specific physical locations, and are situated along the path of the spinal column and head.

We can help to strengthen the energy of the heart by meditating on the heart chakra area and engaging in practices to support and heal any trauma—physical, energetic or metaphysical—the heart area has sustained. This can done for other chakra areas as well. All chakras can be affected by pain and trauma of any kind.

For Bhakti purposes, the practices suggested here focus on the energy of the heart, which, in all types of grief, is deeply affected. The feelings of the heart, the knowledge of the heart and the heart's intelligence are centered on the fourth chakra, *Anahata*, the heart chakra. In grief, our hearts often feel closed, heavy; we may experience pain in that area in different forms. The entire chest area may be sensitive and painful, sore and tender. These sensations may extend outward to the arms and hands. The sensations may be sharp or dull, throbbing or buzzing, stabbing or clenching, persistent or intermittent. Sensations of heaviness may occur. You may experience feelings of anxiety in the heart area including fluttering, rapid or irregular heartbeat or, conversely, your heart may feel sluggish and slow. Each person's experience is unique and also uniquely mutable. What you experienced yesterday may not be the same experience you have today. The heart chakra, the energetic field of the heart, is an incredibly powerful and highly sensitive space. Anahata is located in the center of the chest at the sternum.

The following heart-centered mantras, meditations and mudras can help support your heart center and its energy. They may help you to feel more connected to your own heart center as well as to the Source of Love, to your chosen form of the Divine, and to your beloved dead. They may also help to facilitate any healing in the area of the heart that may be required.

Heart light meditation

Come into a comfortable seated position, cross-legged on the floor, or seated in a supportive chair. If you are sitting in a chair, allow your feet to be flat on the floor, knees relaxed. If you are seated on the floor, ensure comfort by sitting on a cushion or folded blanket, placed just beneath the sitting bones.

Let the spine be long and tall, but not stiff. You may wish to roll the shoulders up toward the ears, back and down, creating a more open chest and heart space. Bringing your hands to your heart area, cross the palms over the heart center in svastika, or cross, mudra (see Figure 3.4). With the palms crossed over the heart, begin to connect with your breath.

Gradually deepen the breath, allowing the inhalation and exhalation to be the same length. Bring your attention and awareness to the spaces between the in and out breath; the hold and the pause. Notice the strength and the rhythm of the beat of your heart within those spaces of holding and pausing between breaths. Return your breath to normal whenever you wish, continuing to have a deep awareness of the beating of your heart.

Notice how you are feeling in your heart space and allow what is, to be. Notice the heart's energy. Do you feel warmth, any sense of movement, waves, vibrations, calmness, fluttering, dullness, aching? Simply notice what you sense and feel, knowing that you do not have to change anything. Be aware of your breath, your feelings and any sensations that may occur throughout the meditation. Simply notice and be with what is.

Imagine a flower with many petals at the center of the chest, in your heart space. See the flower first as a bud. Perhaps the bud is tightly closed or just beginning to open. With each breath, see the bloom open a bit further. With each exhalation, imagine a soft, glowing mist of light— white, pink or green—emanating from the flower bud. Allow this mist to enfold you in a safe, supportive and loving embrace. Imagine as you inhale that you breathe this mist into your being, fragrant and nourishing. Inhaling, allow the cooling, refreshing mist to enter into your nostrils, let it flow gently into the lungs and disperse throughout your being. Notice where the mist of light flows in your body. Perhaps it remains in the heart area, perhaps it moves toward your belly, wraps around your torso or spreads outward to your fingers and toes. Simply notice where it goes.

With each exhalation, let the bud of your heart flower open a bit more, releasing its light and fragrance gently with each breath. As your flower blooms, you are held safely within the love of your own heart. You may imagine the light of flower pulsing with each beat of your heart. Allow whatever is, to be. This is your heart meditation. What you see is what is within your own heart. Know that the light of your heart supports and surrounds you fully in a sphere of safety, complete protection and well-being.

You can practice this meditation anytime you wish. When you are ready to end your heart meditation, lower your hands and open your eyes.

Mudras to support the heart center

A *mudra* is an energetic seal which affects, supports and creates specific changes in our physical, mental, emotional, energetic and spiritual bodies. *Hasta* mudras are those formed by the hands. You may choose to take a hasta mudra while meditating, combined with chant or mantra repetition, while holding a posture in asana practice, when you are sitting in a meeting, standing in a grocery store line, sitting in a waiting room before an appointment or just while sitting and relaxing, watching television, talking to a friend or as you are dropping off to sleep. You can benefit from a mudra anytime, anywhere, any place when your hands, or hand, depending on whether you need one or both for any particular mudra, are free.

Some mudras may feel more comfortable to you than others. Each of the hand mudras presented here help to specifically support the heart, the energies of the heart and Anahata, the heart chakra. As with everything in this book, please make use of the things that feel and seem useful to you and leave others that don't seem to resonate. You may also find that certain mudras appeal for a particular period of time in your life and then they do not. This is all fine.

Mritsamjivani mudra

Mritsamjivani mudra, also known as *apan vayu* mudra, translates in English as "life-saving gesture," and directly supports the overall health of the heart. The mudra helps to regulate blood pressure and to improve circulation. For those suffering from pain in the heart and chest area, or changes in blood pressure following any kind of grief or loss, this mudra is highly recommended. Those not dealing with grief, but who have heart concerns, blood pressure and circulatory problems may also benefit from this mudra. Many believe this mudra can literally save a person's life after a heart attack and can heal the heart of chronic disease on all levels. Energetically and spiritually, this mudra encourages self-care and deep inner reflection.

To form the mudra (Figure 3.5), bring the tip of the index finger to the base of the thumb. Touch the tips of the middle and ring fingers to the tip of the thumb. Extend the little finger outward.

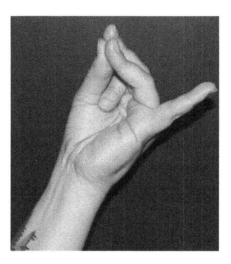

Figure 3.5 Mritsamjivani/Apan vaya mudra.

To apply mritsamjivani mudra, form the mudra with both hands and allow the hands to rest lightly on the thighs as you sit comfortably. The hands may be separate, with a hand resting atop each thigh, or you may choose to bring the hands together, crossing or otherwise joining the little fingers as is comfortable for you, bringing the fingernails of the middle and ring fingers of both hands together to touch lightly. You may hold the mudra in the lap or at the heart center (Figure 3.6).

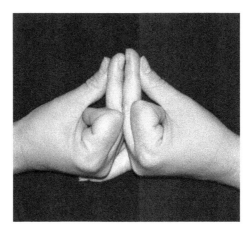

Figure 3.6 Mritsamjivani/Apan vaya mudra at the heart center.

It is suggested that the mudra be held from 5 to 45 minutes as is comfortable. As you hold the mudra, notice any feelings which may arise, particularly those which may be centered in the area of the chest. You may experience lightness, spaciousness, an energetic or emotional softening of the heart center. You may feel movement of the heart energy as the vortex, the whirling motion of the chakra. Each person's experience is individual. You may wish to write about your experiences with this or any mudra in your journal, tracking the use of each mudra and any thoughts, experiences or changes that may occur with your mudra practice.

Padma and sampata mudras

Padma mudra, the gesture of the lotus flower, directly opens Anahata, the heart chakra. Padma is the Sanskrit word for lotus. The lotus begins its journey as a small seed buried within a shallow, murky body of water. As it grows, the roots hold fast to the cool darkness of the muddy bottom while the stem reaches toward the warmth and light above. The bud breaks the surface of the water and opens into an exquisite flower, completely unmarred by the murkiness from which it arises. The flower is greatly revered and serves as an apt metaphor for the human condition due to its humble beginnings and the ultimate radiant beauty of its blossoming. Without the muddy, dark depths which nurture the flower, its flawless beauty would never rise. Because of this, the lotus is sacred in both Hinduism and Buddhism, representing enlightenment, wisdom, purity of heart, pure Love and True knowledge.

The Goddess Lakshmi is closely associated with the lotus flower and is the embodiment of love. It is believed that through the love of Lakshmi our spirits are able to join with the Divine. The Goddess Saraswati is also linked to the image of the lotus blossom as she often appears seated upon a white lotus, representative of perfect and divine knowledge. Her image and powers are also connected to water, where the lotus grows, and which symbolizes creative power, unconscious knowing, inspiration, imagination and the unstoppable flow of cosmic unfolding. Both Goddesses can help us move through the changes of grief, helping the bereaved to open our hearts to love, to new growth and learning, as well as to the realization of deep truths and inner knowledge.

Padma mudra increases heart strength, helps to calm the mind from the stress of racing thoughts, and stimulates the body's ability to heal itself by balancing the immune system. It helps us to feel connected when we feel isolated, recharged when we are depleted, treasured when we feel unappreciated. The mudra also ignites spiritual devotion and inner knowledge of truth through the power of Bhakti love, thereby diminishing the grasping nature of ego, attachment and our tendency to identify with anything other than our True Selves.

The concept of identification and non-attachment can be a delicate and sensitive issue for bereaved persons, particularly those struggling with recent or traumatic grief. We rarely believe we would ever want or choose to release any attachments or identifications with our beloved dead. The thought of doing so is often frightening, even offensive. These kinds of feelings are frequently exacerbated by the insistence of others that we *should* and *need* to let go, to move on, to get over exactly the attachments in which we often find deep solace, even when they are painful.

Usually, our deep identifications with and to our beloveds are rooted solidly in who we think and believe we are in the grief-filled present, as well as who we think and believe we were, to them and with them in the past, when they were solidly, bodily here with us in the physical plane. Memories of our experiences, our hopes, our dreams, our beliefs and ideas about the drastically altered present and the vanished potential futures that will never be are incredibly strong identifying connections to which we grasp and hold close. We often believe, consciously or unconsciously, that our held identifications with our beloveds are our only remaining links with or to them. The idea that these identifications, connections or associations might be dismissed, diminished, reduced or removed in any conceivable way is beyond distressing. I understand that this is true for so many in a visceral way. We need these connections.

Many of the connections, identifications and attachments to which we cling serve great purpose in helping us delve deeply into the pain when we need to do so. They assist us in maintaining and creating new kinds of bonds with our beloveds. They help us know that we can go into the pain and we can come out again. They help us to have compassion toward ourselves and others. When grief is allowed to be what it is, coming in and going out like the tides, when our spirits are nurtured, and when love is honored, identifications and attachments, like grief itself, can transmute and transform without effort or force. There is no time limit on this process.

Padma mudra assists in the release of ego beliefs and identifications that no longer serve us. Such beliefs may include those that tell us we cannot be connected unless we remain in the same places and spaces we have always been. Opening to unknown or heretofore unexplored possibilities inherent in the energies of padma mudra supports us in allowing the connection and relationship to our beloveds to bloom further into new growth, beyond what has always been, into what is now, helping us recognize spiritual and energetic bonds that already exist between us and our beloveds, bonds that existed even before we were formed in this physical realm.

The liberation of deeply ingrained thoughts, ideas and patterns of our past which no longer serve us can allow conscious knowledge of the reality of extant union with those we love who reside in non-physical realms. We too in large part also reside in those places—the realms of thought, imagination, emotion, energy and spirit. Mudras work on all of these levels at once. Our physical being, and theirs, is but a small part of who we and they are. The greater part of us exists in non-physical realms. Just because we can't see something does not mean it's not there. The assistance padma mudra offers is gentle and loving, never violent or forced. All it requires is that we be open to the possibility that we may hold beliefs and identifications that are not serving us, or our relationships to loved ones, living or dead, and that we allow the energies of the mudra to open and support the expansion and growth of heart, mind and spirit.

To form padma mudra (Figure 3.7), begin in anjali mudra with the hands at heart center. Moving the elbows closer to the ribcage, allow this movement to push the hands outward and upward a bit, so that the thumbs are not pressing into the breastbone. Keeping the heels of the palms together, allow the fingers to open, spreading out and upward, into the shape of a blooming flower. The thumbs and little fingers may remain touching or they may be apart, every blooming lotus is different.

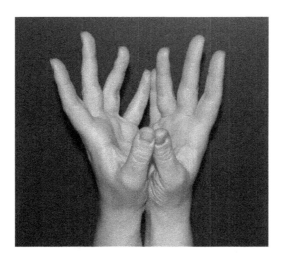

Figure 3.7 Padma mudra.

To apply the mudra, hold your bloom in front of the heart, allowing the belly and chest to soften. The eyes may be closed or gazing toward the center of the bloom. Visualize your lotus blossom in any color you wish. Imagine that a beam of pure radiance emanates from the center of your lotus upward, connecting your heart energy to the Heart of the Source. Allow this radiance to flow through you like a river of pure Love and Knowledge. Know that the radiance of this Love joins you and your loved one eternally. You are also connected with all of creation and the Source of all creation. You are One.

You may also choose to form padma mudra directly from another mudra, *samputa* mudra, meaning vessel or bud. Shifting the mudra from bud to blooming can deepen the mudra practice and is a lovely gesture of growth and opening.

To form samputa mudra (Figure 3.8), bring the hands to the heart center, once again beginning in anjali mudra. From anjali mudra, separate the palms, keeping thumbs, sides of the palms and fingertips touching, to create a hollow space in the center of the palms, forming a bud shape. The bud is samputa mudra, whose energy helps to balance all five elements (Earth, Air, Fire, Water and Ether) throughout the koshas. Samputa mudra reduces mental and emotional suffering, directs our focus inward, and symbolizes inner potential as well as the gateway to the True Self.

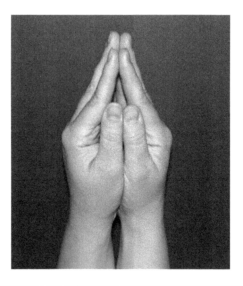

Figure 3.8 Samputa mudra.

Holding this mudra, bring your awareness to the openness between your palms, letting your hands gently and reverently hold the space. Cain and Revital Carroll, authors of *Mudras of India* (2012), beautifully direct the practitioner of samputa mudra to, "hold this space delicately, as if carrying a baby bird"(p.209). You may wish to imagine the pure possibility represented by that lovingly held space. Directing your attention between your palms, visualize your own potential swirling in the gently held space. Perhaps yours is of pure light, or maybe a malleable ball of rich clay, a dancing spark of flame, a bottomless blue sea, a swirling planetary sphere or a star-filled galaxy within an infinite field of quantum space. The jewel within your lotus is yours alone.

It is recommended to hold samputa mudra from 5 to 45 minutes. From samputa mudra, you may choose to allow your bud to open, blooming into padma mudra as you wish, also holding padma mudra anywhere from 5 to 45 minutes.

For both mudras, allow the breath to be easeful, centered in the belly, and the heart center to be soft. As your bud slowly opens with each breath, you may wish to imagine the growth and expansion of your envisioned potential seeping out of the bud with each exhalation. You may wish to imagine with each inhalation, sparks and particles, streams or rivulets of your own potential for growth coming into your being with the breath. You may choose to allow this pure potential to flow in, around and throughout your energetic and subtle bodies, centering on your heart space. Allow it to form a sphere of protection and comfort around you. Allow your potential to move in whatever way feels good and right to you in the moment of the breath. When you feel complete with the practice, release the mudra, take a few centering breaths and notice how you feel. You may wish to write about your experiences in your journal or record them in another medium through art or by talking with a trusted friend or support person.

Anahata chakra mudra

Anahata means "un-struck," which we can think of as a reference to the silence in the openness of the human heart. It's what we feel when the presence of a love so deep, so wide, so expansive and open fills us so that we are unable, and have really no need, to find words to describe it. When we can sit in comfortable, companionable and loving silence with another, when we can gaze deeply into the eyes of one whose heart we know so well that no words are needed to fill the space, this is what is meant by unstruck. No sound, no words. The word also reflects the truest nature of the heart which, regardless of pain, injuries, heartache, grief and sorrow, holds at its deepest center, the energy that is stronger than any hurt it might sustain. A friend described this feeling as that spacious, joyful melting we feel when we see a kitten playing or hear a baby laughing. It's the open, relaxed feeling we experience when our laughter with a dear friend subsides. It's how we feel when we witness something so beautiful that our breath is taken away because our heart space has swollen so that our lungs don't have proper space to expand. These moments are those of the unstruck heart, when the silent reverberation speaks directly to our center.

Imagine the pure, trusting love of a heart that has never been hurt, an unbroken, unbeaten, unstruck heart. This is the nature of the energy of the heart chakra. It's true that our hearts get broken, we are hurt and our hearts feel that pain. But that is not the true nature of the heart. It isn't that we are meant to never experience hardship, pain, sorrow or fear, but rather that the nature of the heart allows us to feel, experience and to move through the pain. And moreover, it can allow the pain to move through *us*, without shutting down our ability to love further, more than we imagined we ever could again. The true nature of the heart is to accept, allow, support and facilitate experiences of joy, peace, compassion, contentment, happiness and deep love. *Anahata chakra*, open and free of blocks, can help us know those states—including after, during, in spite of and even as a result of, experiences that bring deep sorrow, pain and grief. Anahata chakra mudra can help facilitate the opening of the energy center from which that power of love rises.

This mudra, which may seem complicated at first, is powerful, and is used to directly open the heart center. It uses the energies of all the fingers to represent each element, encouraging the energetic balance of the elements within the koshas. The thumbs represent fire; index fingers, air; the little fingers, water. These stretch outward while the middle and ring fingers, representing the elements of Ether and Earth respectively, interlock in the center of the mudra. The configuration of joints and fingers creates a *yantra*, a sacred visual symbol, and in totality, represents the essence of possibility. The shape itself, representing the gateway to the heart, allows the practitioner to visualize the potential of the heart's capacity for compassion and love. This mudra also helps to regulate breathing, bring emotional balance, improve overall heart health and acts to increase all of the practitioner's healing abilities.

To form the mudra (Figure 3.9), place the right ring finger in the web of the index and middle fingers of the left hand. Crossing the left ring finger over the right, place it in the web of the index and middle fingers of the right hand. Curl the two middle fingers downward and over the ring fingers, locking them in place. The two middle fingers will be touching at the first and possibly second knuckles, depending on your fingers. Touch the tips of the index fingers, thumbs and little fingers to each other and extend outward.

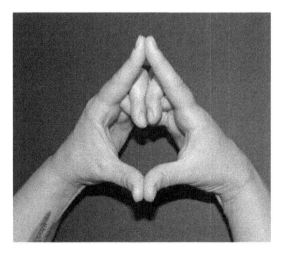

Figure 3.9 Anahata mudra.

To apply the mudra, hold at the heart center while seated in a comfortable position. Hold the mudra anywhere from 5 to 45 minutes. Allow the gaze to be soft, looking toward the center of the mudra. Notice the heart-shape the fingers have formed in the center of the mudra. When you feel calm and centered, close your eyes. Allow them to soften, imagine the eyeballs dropping backward and down, allowing your vision to shift to an inward gaze. Allow that gaze to focus inwardly on your heart center. Imagine your gaze can see behind and beyond all pain, sorrow and heartbreak you have experienced, not only from your current grief, but all grief, all pain, all harm, and hurt since you came into this body at your physical birth. Imagine that behind all of the ache and the hurt, there is an unending expanse of unbroken, unhurt, unconditional, unstruck love. This love exists eternally for you, your experiences, your loved ones, your family, your friends, for acquaintances, for strangers, even for those who may have hurt you in the past, not knowing the Truth of their own Self.

Rumi wrote,

> Out beyond the ideas of wrongdoing and
> rightdoing, there is a field.
> Meet me there.
> When the soul lies down in that grass, the
> world is too full to talk about.
> Ideas, language, even the phrase each
> other, doesn't make any sense.

(1997, p.98)

This is the field of the unstruck heart. This is the field in which your original, unchanged, unstruck heart can speak freely to you in its own voice. Imagine the field, your field, covered in soft, spring green grass. The color of this grass is the restful and nourishing green of the light of Anahata chakra. Lie back into that softness. Rest a while, and allow the love of your own heartfield to hold you. Notice what you see in your field. Sit up if you like; still you are held. Notice the sky, the clouds, the quality and character of the sun's light and warmth, and whether there is anything or anyone else in the field. You may be able to sense the presence of their energy or you may visualize these others there with you. Your beloveds, animal or insect guides, beings of light or energy, other plant life, the presence of the elements: Air, Fire, Water, Earth, Ether. Permit whatever is simply to be. Let the nourishing, loving, supportive space of your heartfield reveal itself to you. Bask in this experience as long as you wish. When you are ready, open your eyes, release the mudra, take a few cleansing breaths, place your hands on the Earth or the floor if you need grounding. Notice how you are feeling. You may wish to write about your experiences in your journal or record them in another creative way.

Abhaya hrdaya mudra

Abhaya hrdaya mudra is the courageous heart mudra. Going through the pain of grief is one of the most discouraging, disheartening experiences imaginable. In grief, we can all use a bit of extra courage. Courage gives us the ability to face and move through pain, uncertainty, fear and hardship. Courage does not change the situation, but it can help us withstand it. You did not choose this, but here you are. There are days when it seems that every ounce of effort you can muster is required simply to get out of bed. There are times when it seems to take all your strength and energy to open your eyes, to face the day, to face the mirror, to face the empty house, to face the rest of the world as it moves on and on, to face the pain of your beloved's absence. Again. And then again. And again the next day. The next week, month and year. And again the year after that. Thinking of a lifetime without them can be petrifying.

You might try forming abhaya hrdaya mudra before getting out of bed each day, before getting out of the car to go in to work, before going into a grocery store or other public place, before any activity that you know will trigger memories, grief and pain. It will not make grief go away, but perhaps your strength can be buoyed a bit and your energy lifted, which may help you get through a difficult undertaking, whatever it might be.

Abhaya hrdaya mudra nurtures the heart as well as the lungs—which are greatly affected by grief. In Traditional Chinese Medicine, grief is the emotion of the lungs. Many grieving people have the sensation of being unable to breathe fully; sometimes you might unconsciously hold your breath until you find yourself gasping for air, not even realizing you weren't breathing. I remember that sensation well, being unexpectedly startled by the sudden need for air, as if I had been underwater, my lungs hurting from the lack of breath. This can be jarring, but is a common occurrence for many when swimming in the vast sea of grief.

The primary way that *prana*, the universal life force known in Chinese Medicine as Qi (pronounced *chee*), and in Japanese traditions as Ki (pronounced *kee*), enters our being is through the breath. It comes into our lungs with each inhalation and is dispersed throughout the physical body as well as throughout the other koshas as appropriate. Oxygen is carried through the physical body by the circulatory system, but prana can and does permeate all the bodies, physical as well as subtle. Not only does prana, energizing, life-giving force, move throughout, but it can be directed to the specific places we send it. This is what yoga teachers are talking about when they say strange things like, "Breathe into your side body (or your intercostal muscles, or your hamstrings, or your hip flexors)…" or, "Direct the breath to the place where you feel your edge." We can tell the prana where to go to help us in the places we need it most. When the lung function is compromised, reduced or out of balance due to nearly anything—stress, illness, emotional imbalance, and, of course, grief and sadness—our ability to receive, as well as direct, prana is also thereby diminished.

Abhaya hrdaya mudra also supports the digestive system. Interestingly, the large intestine is the partner organ to the lungs in the system of Chinese Medicine, and acts as the yang to the yin of the lungs. In grief, digestive function can be greatly impaired. Each person experiences these effects individually, but a grieving person's appetite and the ability to tolerate or digest food is almost always affected, therefore resulting in further imbalance and undesirable effects to the rest of the body's systems.

Emotionally, abhaya hrdaya mudra helps to bring a sense of calm and strength. It reduces fragmented thoughts and restores a sense of wholeness to weakened or scattered energy. It also helps to reduce nightmares and soothe a troubled mind. A powerful energy conductor, this mudra is supportive and restorative when you feel exhausted, fearful, devitalized, nervous, and out of control.

To form abhaya hrdaya (Figure 3.10), cross the wrists at the chest, with the backs of the hands touching, right hand closest to the body. Interlock the index, middle and little fingers. Connect the tips of the ring fingers to the tips of the thumbs on both hands, forming two rings.

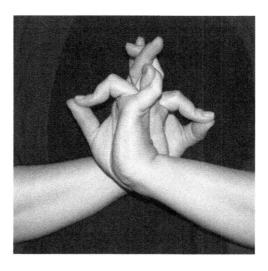

Figure 3.10 Abhaya hrdaya mudra.

To apply the mudra, bring the formed mudra to the chest, pulling downward gently but firmly, rooting the mudra at the base of the sternum. This mudra allows energy to descend from the head to the lower body, creating a sense of deep groundedness and security in body and mind. Notice any sensations you experience while holding this mudra. Follow the descent and movement of energy as it flows through the koshas. Breathing normally, hold the mudra for 5 to 45 minutes.

As always, with this or any mudra or other practice, you may wish to write about your experiences in your journal, or record them in another medium through art, or by talking with a trusted friend or support person.

Suggestions to cultivate a Bhakti practice

- Begin your day with devotional practices, daily meditation, daily ritual or *puja* (prayer ceremony).

- Create altars and shrines.

- Tend and maintain your altar or shrine, with fresh flowers, cleaning, arranging, adding or removing various elements on the altar, removing any depleted offerings.

- Chant the name of your chosen deity or another mantra of your choice.

- Sing daily. Singing opens the heart. Sing your favorite hymn or song of love, practice *kirtan* (traditional devotional chanting of the names of God), write your own devotional and/or love songs.

- Allow daily times of prayer and contemplation or ritual acts such as lighting a candle.

- Write your own prayer that you read and speak daily.

- Write love letters to your beloved.

- Practice daily asana poses, such as *surya namaskar* (sun salute) as a devotional offering to your chosen deity or in honor of your beloved dead.

- Visit holy or spiritual sites where devotional practices take place.

- Cry freely if you are so moved. To cry is to express love and longing. It is a prayer and a devotional practice.

Chapter 4

Tantra Yoga

The Path of Transformation

The very definition of yoga as union encourages the grieving person that he or she can connect with something other than the pain that isolates us. This fundamental axiom gives hope and provides tools to assist in bridging the seeming chasms between us and our beloved dead. The same tools can help us to feel less separate from others, from nature and from Spirit. Yoga teaches that we are perfect and whole *as we are*. Tantra yoga does this by letting us know that, simply because we are part of this world, we are therefore part of the Divine All. You are enough—perfectly and exactly as you are; in pain, in joy, in peace, in grief. It is in the recognition of this Truth that we can be transformed.

The truth of all yogic paths is that ultimately there is no division between the Divine All and us. The Tantric path's major distinction from the other branches of yoga is the direct focus on the radiant power and supreme function of the Divine feminine, the energy of the Goddess, as inherent in all form and matter, movement and energy. All spiritual paths that have a direct focus on the Divine feminine are, in essence, Tantric paths. These include all Goddess paths: Wicca and other various forms of paganism, Native American spirituality, Buddhist Tantric practices, Taoist Tantra, many tribal, shamanic and indigenous paths, as well as the spiritual paths of ancient cultures of Rome, Greece, Egypt, Babylon, Mesopotamia, Sumer, Polynesia and ancient Europe.

Tantra yoga is a highly misunderstood and misinterpreted branch of yoga, particularly in Western culture, where it is often thought of as a path that focuses solely on sexuality. While Tantric practices and rituals can include sexual acts, sexuality is only part of a rich Tantric tradition. Traditionally, there are two basic schools of Tantra. Some practitioners and scholars refer to these as the "right-handed" and the "left-handed" paths, others refer to Tantra's different aspects in terms of color: white, pink and red Tantra.

The right-handed path focuses primarily on deep individual inner work—mantra, mudra, meditation and other visionary kinds of practices. The left-handed path includes meditative practices as well as rituals involving sexuality. Historically, left-handed paths also included rituals in burial or crematory grounds, sometimes involving skulls, bones or ashes to accentuate the importance of understanding the intricate dance of life and death as well as secret rites said to result in the acquisition of magical or supernatural powers. White Tantra corresponds essentially with the right-handed path, while red and pink Tantric practices are compatible with the left-handed path. Regardless of the chosen path, all of Tantra is about the eternal flow of creative energy and the essential non-duality of all. Tantra teaches that humanity, our very beings, our bodies, hearts, minds and spirits contain all possibilities of reality and existence.

The way of the Goddess

Most people with even a passing awareness of Eastern religions, particularly of Hinduism, know that Goddesses are worshipped and revered throughout Asia. Practices and sacred texts of Tantra, which first emerged around the sixth century CE, fully recognize and revere the Divine feminine principle as the primal force of all power, creation and evolution throughout the universe and all time. Tantra teaches and aids us in the realization that the physical world in which we live is filled with and entirely comprised of Divine energy and power. In the yogic tradition, this power is the feminine force known as *Shakti*, which helps us learn to be free of the illusion of our own separateness from the world around us. It also gives the Tantric practitioner, a *tantrika*, or *tantrik* in the masculine form, the tools to make life in this world richer and more bountiful in all manner of thinking and being. These tools can also help the tantrika to live a more productive, peaceful life filled with wonder, beauty and personal power with deep connection to Spirit and the Divine All. This includes lives that are touched by, even suffused with grief, trauma and pain. Tantra includes *all* experiences of humanity as part of the Divine experience. For the tantrik, all of life, as well as death, is sacred and worthy of honor. This truth is validation of the myriad experiences and expressions of life, including grief.

The word "Tantra" itself describes the path beautifully. The Sanskrit language is multilayered and each word, as well as roots of words, can have multiple meanings. The word *tantra* is formed by the joining of two parts. *Tan* means to expand, to extend, to stretch, to develop. It also means to weave. Imagine the combined energies and experiences of us all being woven together on a Divine loom. Picture the threads of existence being layered, the warp and the weft of the fibers of each heart and mind, layering, stretching and extending further and further into the ever-expanding tapestry of one creation. The suffix *tra* meaning "tool" or "instrument" is the loom on which the creation is formed and also the tools the tantrika uses to participate in creation. Tantra, and yoga overall, provides technological tools based on Divine science to help us better function in life, to be more peaceful and more productive.

With its focus on physical and sensual experiences of the now, Tantra may seem to be different from other branches of yoga, which seem to encourage us to move beyond the physical to a place of spirit, elevated above and beyond our corporeal existence. The concept of the whole of the physical world as *maya*, illusion, seems to communicate that ultimately what occurs in the physical realm is not what actually matters. Is this physical life a trick or a test? Merely something to be gotten through until the end when we are liberated? Are we meant to muck our way through the physical world and its sufferings, with minds and hearts fixed on the spiritual realm beyond until we eventually become "enlightened" enough to rise above and escape it all?

Tantra teaches that it is not the physical world that is unreal or illusory, but only our own unknowing; the false belief that we are separate from God/ dess. We are One always; including when we are in physical form—living, learning, working, playing, laughing, longing, grieving, growing—in the physical world. The physical plane is not lifetime after lifetime of drudgery to be slogged through until the long-awaited day of liberation when we are finally rewarded with freedom from this painful world and its projections of false reality. No. Tantra teaches that liberation is here and now; in these bodies, in this world, in this life as well as beyond. We are already liberated. We need only see it.

The Divine physics of Mother Nature

All matter is essentially an arrangement of condensed energy in material form. The Vedic seers called this essential creative energy *prakriti*, which means, literally, "nature"; it is also translated to mean "energy." This energy is also known as Shakti and is a feminine force. Shakti power is everything in existence. All that we see, feel, touch and experience in the material universe exists because of Shakti and is made of Shakti. Tantra acknowledges and focuses on this Goddess energy that gives rise to all life, all movement, all change, all pleasure, all pain, all inspiration, all evolution, all creation, all destruction. She is everything that is physically and energetically manifest. The word "matter" is derived from the Latin *mater*, meaning mother. She is all matter, all sound, all light and the absence of all of these. She is every animal, mineral and vegetable. She is Earth, Air, Fire, Water and Ether. She is every atom of every element and the space between them. She is Mother Nature, the energy of weather, the changing of the seasons, the turning of the planets and the stars, the tidal movements of the ocean and the beating of our hearts. She is birth, death and everything in between.

The fundamental difference in Tantra practice from all other branches of yoga is the primary focus on the Goddess as the force that underlies, creates and maintains all that we see and know, and the belief that we don't have to do anything or go anywhere to experience that power and connection because She is here with us, in us, as us, all the time. She dwells in the now, the physical. She is the power that is responsible for the ability you have to think about your own ideas and experiences related to what you are reading in this very moment. She is that which allows the connection between you and me that is happening right now, though we may have never met. We are in this moment connected. We are One.

In the Hindu pantheon of many gods and goddesses, all of whom are various aspects of the unchanging Shiva/Shakti Absolute, the masculine and feminine faces of the Supreme Being—it is known that the male gods cannot act without their female counterparts. They can only be and witness. It is the feminine that creates and acts.

In the Tantric view, the concepts of masculine and feminine are very different than those held by Western cultures. The masculine power, the witnessing awareness, the pure consciousness of Shiva is by its very nature, passive, while the energetic, creative, swirling, ever expanding, ever-moving energy of Shakti is active. Both need the other. Without Shakti, Shiva would be content to sit in His pure state of awareness, all-knowing, all-seeing, never moving, never changing, never creating, never engaging, simply being. Without Shiva, the kinetic powerful energy of Shakti would be unable to find stability, the matter that her creative energy generates cannot hold together without the aspect of His ultimate focus, consciousness and awareness. In their joining, all manner of creation can form and hold. With this, the belief is also that every creation in all of the cosmos has a witnessing consciousness, part Him, part Her. His peaceful witness consciousness is always there, gazing out from within Her living, dancing, vibrating molecules.

The holy seers of Vedic sciences, at least 5000 years ago, and based on some accounts closer to 10,000 years ago, saw and intuited things that through the findings of modern science we know to be true today. They knew that all matter is condensed energy; they knew that all matter is made of the same star dust. We also know through quantum physics, and with the use of tools that allow us to see beyond and beneath what our human senses allow, that every single thing in existence is made of atoms all of which are in movement, vibrating at various frequencies. Some forms of matter have a slower vibratory rate, like rocks and minerals, but they vibrate nonetheless, while other things like plants and animals vibrate at higher rates. All of these scientific concepts and more were written about by ancient Vedic scientists thousands of years ago. This system holds that all matter has intelligence and consciousness, and exists only due to the merging of the energies of Shiva and Shakti. Each of us individually is a melding of Shiva and of Shakti.

By consciously tapping into our abilities to experience ourselves as Shiva and as Shakti, we can experience more fully both the physical and non-physical realms, as well as better understand our Oneness with the Divine All. Because we are firmly rooted in the world of the physical, which is Shakti manifest, we can consciously offer our daily existence and experiences in the world as ritual. By honoring the presence of the Goddess, becoming more aware of Her energy within and around us, we are helped to realize our fundamental connection to creation.

For grieving people this can be a vital and affirming experiential path. In grief we so often feel disconnected, isolated and alone. Many grieving people have experiences of feeling betrayed: by God or religion, by their own bodies, by loved ones, living and dead, and frequently by the world that continues to go on as if nothing has happened, when the most precious thing we hold close is somehow, insensibly, irretrievably gone. It makes no sense. Our bodies often feel numb; we can feel completely removed from the world around us. Because of this disconnection, our energy feels low or, sometimes, extremely high and out of control. We may experience sensations—physical and energetic—of extreme discomfort, and feel a lack of ability to be soothed by, or connected to, anything, ever again.

Tantra can bring the comforting support of the Mother to our broken hearts and help us to feel not only Her power, but our own. Who has not wished at the lowest points of confusion, helplessness and vulnerability to be soothed and held by an unconditionally loving Mother? Tantra can help us experience that love and gain power from the knowledge that She is with us and in us. Her love is unending, all-encompassing. Tantric practices provide tools to help the bereaved to feel and sense the power and the presence of our beloved dead in and around us as well, for they never leave us.

The principle of physics which tells us that energy can never die nor be destroyed can help us to understand in a very basic way the truth of the knowledge of the Vedas. Energy cannot be destroyed. It only changes form. When we are alive, the energy that moves our bodies is a combination of prana, the life force, and Shakti, the creative, manifesting force of literally everything in existence, including things that are invisible to the human eye. Once a person dies, pranic energy no longer exists in the body. At death, the physical body ceases to function as living matter and neither requires nor uses prana. The body is the vehicle which holds, uses and manifests the energy which moves it. The yogic and the tantric view is that this energy continues to exist.

Recall the Jnana chapter where we explored the contemplation of the question, "Who Am I?" Jnana teaches us that we are not our bodies. Knowing this, where then do we go when the body no longer functions? The energy of who we are never dies. This energy is dispersed or dispatched elsewhere. It is released from the body that ceases to function as a living human and the energy continues on. None of us really ever dies; our energy merely changes form. As a bereaved mother I don't say this lightly. I understand that, even with full and total acceptance of and belief in the concept of never-dying energy, this in no way replaces the concrete experience of seeing, hearing, touching, feeling and holding our beloveds as they were in their bodies on this physical plane. I know that. But here we are.

Consider this: Just as energy never dies, love never dies. Love is pure energy. Because energy cannot be destroyed, we can know that the energy that once moved their bodies, the energy that shined forth from our beloveds, in whatever form they took, for however long, in physical and scientific fact, still exists. The love that connects us to them also exists. Tantra gives us tools to better understand the ways that energy changes; how it moves and how it impacts the physical as well as energetic, emotional, mental and spiritual realms in which we reside. It involves noticing, locating, following, shifting, changing, creating, building and sharing energy within and around our environments, our bodies, and throughout the koshas.

The system of the koshas

In working with Tantra, we are working with energy and the way it moves throughout our bodies. To understand this, we must understand the system of the koshas (Figure 4.1). Kosha literally means sheath. The five koshas conceal, and in many ways, also reveal, the True Self. The sheaths of the koshas move from the densest layer, the physical, to the most subtle inner layer of the True Self.

In yogic traditions, "subtle" is something which cannot be seen by the physical eye, but which is nonetheless very real. Each kosha affects the others. Those nearest each other have more direct effect on neighboring koshas. Many yoga teachers explain the koshas with the metaphor of a glass hurricane lantern. As the flame burns, eventually the inside of the globe becomes covered in layers of soot and the inner flame visually dampened. When the grime is cleared away, the flame shines forth brightly. The flame has never changed; it was always as bright. Our True Selves are the flame. With yogic practices the koshas can become clearer, each more in harmony with the other. When this occurs, our inner flame shines out more clearly. Another metaphor of the sheaths of the koshas is the image of Russian nesting dolls, *matryoshkas*. Each doll is nestled inside and beside the next until you reach the center where the final doll rests.

Each kosha name contains the Sanskrit *maya*, which means illusion, or more accurately, *delusion*. This does not mean that the koshas are not real. It means that things appear to be one way, but in truth and reality, are actually another. Maya, of necessity, creates for us highly convincing delusions. If not for maya, life—or death—would not exist as we know it.

The root of the Sanskrit "maya" is *ma* which means "to measure" and also "to make" or "to create." It is also thought by scholars to be the root of the Latin *mater*, "mother," which also relates to the word *matter*. This maya that Shakti creates measures out the indivisible Infinite into finite and seemingly separate forms. In *Awakening Shakti* (2013, p.38), author Sally Kempton writes, "When Shakti is manifesting as the deluding force of Maya, it's difficult to see the hidden connections between ourselves and the rest of the physical world. It's even harder to recognize the invisible forms of the cosmic powers, even though they live inside and around us."

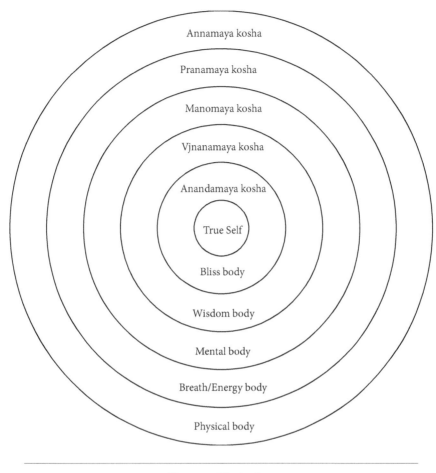

Figure 4.1 The koshas.

It is the nature of Shakti to conceal Herself and so She does throughout all of existence. There are layers upon layers of concealment. There is also much concealed in the maya of grief. This is what many bereaved learn as we live day after day, year after year without our beloveds. We can learn that grief conceals great gifts and becomes something we would never choose to part with in this life. Even if we would never choose the circumstances that wrought it, we would not give it up. Do we continue to miss and love and wish for our loved ones to be with us? Yes. But when we see that grief is love, why would we ever want to give it up? It becomes a comforter, a companion in its constancy. Lacking the ability to change the fact of death, finding sanctuary within grief can be, like the power of Shakti, profoundly transformative.

Grief in itself is neither positive nor negative. It is the result of the loss of a precious treasure. It is the normal and natural reaction to the loss of something precious. The pain inherent in this is axiomatic, but that does not change the nature of grief as highly mutable. This is one of the secrets concealed within the raw, searing, hateful pain of new and traumatic grief. It feels like we ourselves may die from the pain. But we do not. Then, somehow, we come to a place where we can learn to begin to sit with our grief, we can learn to make a companion of our grief. Grief is a multilayered experience and affects us as individuals uniquely on every level of being. The koshas are those levels of our being. Each one is impacted by the experience of deep grief. The more traumatic the experience of grief, the more protracted and extensive the effect on the koshas. As we begin to work with energy, having a basic knowledge of the koshas, what they are, how they function, and how they are impacted by grief, will be useful.

Tantra involves expression, recognition, movement and balancing of energy through the koshas using mindfulness, practice and ritual. The system of the koshas is relevant to all branches and all practices of yoga, whether we are practicing asana, meditation, contemplation, inquiry, service, ritual or other aspects of yoga. And, of course, because we know that they are not really separate, when one layer of our being is affected, all are. The idea of separateness that is actually Oneness is particularly well illustrated in and through the koshas.

Meditations on the koshas

Each kosha description is followed by a meditation on that kosha. The kosha meditations can be done individually, kosha by kosha, or together as one long continuous meditation. Once you become comfortable with noticing and giving attention to the koshas, you can tune into each of them more easily in your practices or any time during the day to check in with how you are feeling and functioning on all levels.

To begin your meditations on the koshas, turn off phones and other electronic devices that could create a distraction. Find a comfortable spot, on a chair or on the floor. If you sit on the floor, you may wish to use a cushion or folded blanket to support the sitting bones and to allow the hips to be comfortable. If you choose to sit in a chair, let your feet be flat on the floor. Allow your hands to rest in your lap or on your knees in a comfortable position. Allow your spine to be long and tall, but not stiff. Roll your neck from side to side to release tension. Take a few deep, cleansing breaths, focusing on expanding your abdomen. Allow your breathing to return to normal.

If you like, make a ritual of the kosha meditations in which you honor your body, the koshas in all their functions, appreciating and honoring what each one does for us. You may wish to light a candle, play soft music or say a prayer or chant a sacred mantra before beginning.

The first kosha—annamaya kosha

As *anna* means "food," the annamaya kosha is literally the sheath made of food. You actually are what you eat. Annamaya kosha is our physical body which is created from the nutrients we bring into it. Annamaya kosha is everything that exists of us, all that we can see, feel, touch and hear, including internal organs and systems, in the physical world. Take your hand and connect it to some part of your body—thigh, arm, belly, breast, knee. Run your hands through your hair, give your own neck a massage, rub your temples. Using both arms, give your whole upper body a hug. This is annamaya kosha. Skin, muscle, fatty tissue, bone, ligament, tendon, hair, sweat, tears, blood, teeth—all the pieces and parts of the tangible, physical body are annamaya kosha.

In classical yoga, many of the practices, particularly those of Hatha, are meant to make life more comfortable in the physical body. Healthy, more flexible, stronger bodies make for fewer obstacles, allowing for deeper abilities in practices that create access to the more subtle koshas. Tantric practices, as well as Hatha yoga practices, bring, encourage and create intense awareness and exploration of our physical bodies and how they interact with the other koshas.

The entirety of annamaya kosha is affected by grief. Like a weight that presses down and into the physical body, grief can impact and disturb all biological rhythms and processes. Appetite is almost always affected—eating too much or having no appetite at all, fluctuating between these possibilities. Digestive problems—upset stomach, nausea, irritable bowel and more are common. Sleep patterns are disrupted—sleeping more than usual, or not at all, or waking at various times throughout the night. Dreams may come that are frightening and anxiety-provoking. Increased levels of stress hormones create havoc in the brain and the central nervous system where responses of distress and fear are triggered. Intense anxiety and bodily symptoms of panic are common for many grieving people. Because the beloved is dead, the body is plunged into its age-old fight or flight response, as if our very survival depends on theirs.

Physical pain in various body parts, including the arms and the heart area particularly, is common. The everyday weight of grocery bags, a laundry basket or even car keys can seem to weigh a thousand pounds. Fine motor skills may no longer exist for a period. Clumsiness, increased risk of physical accidents, falling, tripping, running into things are commonplace among the bereaved. Depth perception and ability to judge where our bodies are in space are compromised. Extreme fatigue and the inability to rise from the sofa, the bed, the toilet, or the floor are common.

Conversely, inexplicable bouts of manic energy can cause crazed floor pacing at 3 a.m., buzzing with an incomprehensible physical need to somehow move, to dig, to flail, to run, to stomp, to pound; despite bone-deep exhaustion, we can feel driven by energy that feels it must find a release. To sit still can feel like coming out of your skin.

Other common physical signs of grief include dry, itchy, red, burning, stinging, swollen eyes, these may be due to crying and/or lack of sleep. Our very skin can change—texture, color, complexion, sometimes due to dehydration and dryness from lack of drinking enough water, lack of self-care, intense crying, hormonal changes and the havoc being wrought in the body's systems overall. Sensitivity to sensory input such as loud noises and crowded spaces, bright light, music, the conversation of others, can make all manner of other sights and sounds difficult to tolerate. Visual and auditory input can be incredibly anxiety-provoking. Panic attacks are common among the bereaved, very often when venturing out into the world of the living that goes on as if nothing has happened.

Mothers grieving the death of a baby deal with additional physical symptoms that seem beyond cruel and painful. Breasts swollen and painful with no baby to suckle and feed. Bodies recuperating from the travails of childbirth with no reward of a baby to care for. Hands, arms, heart and womb experiencing the kind of pain akin to phantom limb syndrome, needing to hold and care for the beloved child that is not there. Ears that hear phantom cries of the baby who is loved, missed and desperately wanted. The list of physical changes that are possible in grief is extensive. The physical body is ravaged in so many ways by grief.

Annamaya kosha meditation

Sit in a comfortable position, allowing the spine to be long, but not stiff. Sit in a position that allows the hips and knees to feel relaxed; in a chair or on the floor. For this meditation, you will remove your shoes. Let the hands be relaxed and comfortable. Take a few deep breaths. Roll the neck and head from side to side, releasing tension. You may keep your eyes open or closed, whichever feels more comfortable.

When you are ready, bring your attention to all that is your physical body. This is annamaya kosha. With gentleness and openness, simply notice, see, feel and experience it without judgment. Think for a moment of all the work this body does for you each day. Each movement, each breath, each step; this body takes you from place to place. Upon waking in the morning until going to sleep at night, it works, never ceasing its efforts to carry you through the world as it has done since your birth and as it will up until the very moment of your death.

This body is yours alone. It is the sacred vehicle now holding your spirit. It touches, sees, hears, tastes, experiences, feels and remembers. It eats, sleeps, digests, eliminates and heals itself when it becomes ill or injured. It produces energy by taking nutrients from the foods it takes in, and brings information from the world around you. It allows you experiences of pleasure and alerts you to pain.

Begin simply to notice the physical characteristics and sensations of this body. Notice the space that it occupies, and the edges of its physical boundaries. Notice whether you feel any tension or pain, a sense of comfort or discomfort. Without changing anything at all, simply notice this body that is yours. Begin to cultivate in this moment a sense of gratitude toward this body. Release all judgment in this moment about this body. Simply notice and allow your body to be in this moment.

Without changing anything, move your awareness to the toes, to the soles of the feet, the tops of the feet and to the ankles. Notice what each of these body parts is feeling right now. Is there tension present? Are they relaxed? What, if anything, are the soles of the feet touching right now? Are the feet flexed or pointed? If you wish, move the feet around, rotate the ankles, point the toes and then flex them, wiggle or spread them wide, allow the toes to relax. Notice what varies or shifts with this movement. Are there sounds? Changes in pressure within the joints? Do you notice a release of tension? Squeeze, rub or massage the toes, feet and ankles. What do you notice?

Move your awareness now to the calves, the shins and the knees. Give attention to any sensation there. Are the muscles in this area tight? Are they comfortable? Are they restricted? What do you notice about this part of the body? Feel and touch these parts of your body. Can you feel the bones of the shins? Notice variations in the musculature of the calves and the intricate structure of the knee cap. Feel the soft give of the patellar tendons that cover the knee cap and join shin bones to thigh bones. Send the hands here to rub, caress or massage these areas if you wish. Notice what you feel and experience.

Become aware of your thighs, the meaty muscles covering the femur bones, the largest and strongest bones in the body. Grasp a chunk of each thigh in your hands. Reach around to the hamstrings. Feel how large, long and strong these muscles are. Notice the curvature of the thighs, notice where they are soft, where the skin may be textured. Become aware of the hip joints, are they open or are they tight? In whatever way you are sitting can you open your hips further? However your hips are feeling, whatever position they occupy, simply notice the hips. If you wish, bring your hands to your hips and press downward. Can you feel the hip bones beneath your palms? What is your experience of the flesh that covers these bones? Notice the softness covering hardness. Become aware of the pelvic bowl which houses the reproductive organs, the bladder and the colon. Press your fingers gently into the abdomen being aware of the feel of the tissue there. Bring the awareness to the sitting bones. If you wish, move some of the flesh out of the way so these bones are more easily experienced. Rock slightly side to side, tilt your pelvis front and back. Notice how the bony protrusions hold the weight of the body.

Bring the awareness to the low back, the sacral area, the spine. Allow your hands to move here. Notice what you feel. Become aware of each vertebra, one stacking upon the next, each separated by intervertebral discs, absorbing the impact of all movement and weight. If your spine is healthy and you are in no pain, allow the back to round forward, noticing how this changes the sensation. Arch the back, lifting the chest, then allow it to return to a neutral position. Tilt the chin toward the chest and notice the changes and movements of the vertebra of the neck. Tilt the head gently side to side. Notice how the spine holds the weight of the head. If it is comfortable, bring the right hand to the left knee, and allow the spine to twist gently, keeping the natural curvature of the spine intact. Look over the left shoulder as far as is comfortable. Release the twist and bring the left hand to the right knee, repeating this gentle twist on the other side. Release the twist and return to the center with a neutral spine. Notice any changes that you experience.

Bring awareness to the rib cage, which protects so many vital organs: the lungs, the heart, parts of the stomach, the liver and the spleen. Bring the hands to the ribs and explore the physical body in this space. Notice their curve, the shape of the ribs. Taking a deeper, fuller breath, notice how they move when the lungs expand.

Allow the breath to return to normal, bringing hands to heart center, cross your hands over the chest in svastika mudra (see Figure 3.4, page 82). Press into the center of the chest gently, feeling the sternum and the soft tissue that covers it. Bring your attention to the beating of the heart. Become aware in this moment of the never-ending movement of the systems of this body; always moving, always pumping, always working, always producing, always creating.

Allow your awareness, and your hands if you wish, to travel from the heart area to the neck, shoulders and throat. Let the fingers explore this area, noticing the feel of the collarbones, the ropy muscles of the neck, the gentle undulation of the throat as you swallow. Notice what changes in the throat, shoulders or collarbones as you breathe. Bring the hands to the back of the neck and feel the curve of the cervical spine.

Bring the hands to your lap and let them touch and grasp each other. Feel each finger, the nails, the cuticles. Notice each finger and the thumbs, each knuckle, each joint; the radial bones of the hands, the knobby bones of the wrists. Notice the skin of the hands and the palms. Notice and think for a moment of all the hands do for you. All the small and large movements, touching, grasping, eating, picking up, holding, working, scratching, rubbing, feeling, tiny movements and large. Allow each hand to grasp the other at the wrist, the forearms, up the arms to the biceps, triceps, to the shoulders and the deltoid muscles there. Feel the shoulders and again each side of the neck.

With the eyes now gently closed, allow the hands and fingers to explore the face. Imagine that you have never seen this face before and are now, for the first time "seeing" it with your hands only. What do you feel? Notice the softness, the roughness, where there are ridges, where there is space, where there is hair or not. Are there moles, bumps, textures, curves, planes or angles? Allow the fingers to trace the shape of the eyebrows, the curve of the eye sockets, the bridge of the nose, the shape of the lips. Notice the jawbone, the curve and the planes of the cheeks and the cheekbones beneath. Bring the fingers to the temples; give this area a gentle circular massage if you wish. Explore the ears, how the tissue there bends and stretches. Feel and notice each curve of the ear, the softness, notice the sounds that your ears hear as they are explored by your fingers.

Move the hands to the head, noting the curve and the shape of the skull. Bring the hands to the back of the head, feeling the bony ridge at the back, the occipital bone. Allow the hands to move through the hair, noticing its length, its texture. Notice the texture of the skin, the roughness or smoothness. Notice the feeling where there may be no hair on the skull, where hair ends and begins. Note the skin of the head, how loose or how tight it is against the bone. Massage the scalp gently, scratching the head if you wish. Notice the sensations. Allow the fingers to feel the shape of the skull. Place one hand on your forehead and the other on the back of the neck at the base of the skull. Send a "thank you" and a blessing to this body that does so much for you each day of your life.

When you have completed the exploration of annamaya kosha, allow your hands simply to rest in the lap or on the thighs. What do you notice? How do you feel? Releasing judgment, what are your observations? When you are ready to complete this portion of the meditation, bring the hands to the heart center in anjali mudra in gratitude to the physical body.

The second kosha—pranamaya kosha

Pranamaya kosha is the sheath of prana. Many refer to this kosha as the "breath body" and this is somewhat accurate, but prana is not the same as the breath. Breath is vital, that's for sure. If we do not have it, we will die in a matter of minutes. Annamaya kosha cannot function without oxygen for its tissues. Knowing how much we need oxygen for life, we require prana even more. We can survive for several minutes deprived of oxygen; think of holding your breath underwater. Prana does not work the same way. We can direct, hold and move prana, but when it is removed from the body, even for millisecond, a nanosecond, death is immediate. Prana can be increased or decreased, but never leaves the physical body completely until the functions of annamaya kosha cease.

Both breath and prana are greatly affected by the experience of grief. Many grieving people experience the sensation of being unable to breathe fully. Particularly in early grief, many bereaved involuntarily, unknowingly, hold our breath, finding ourselves suddenly gasping for air, not realizing the breath was failing to come in and out of the body like it should. Great sighs and yawns are not uncommon as our bodies try to replenish diminished oxygen as well as pranic energy. As discussed in the chapter on Bhakti, in the practice of abhaya hrdaya mudra, grief and the lungs are intimately connected. Our ability to breathe properly is greatly affected by the physical and energetic changes grief brings. Prana's reduction is due to restricted and shallow breath, the precarious state of annamaya kosha under the physical impact of grief, as well as grief and trauma-related blockages in the chakras, which reside in pranamaya kosha.

Prana reduction can also be related to other factors such as decreased exposure to sunlight, isolation, lack of self-care in diet and exercise, lack of sleep and other long-term sequelae of grief such as stress related illnesses, immune system compromise and myriad psychosocial stressors of grief which greatly influence the energy body. Increasing the intake and levels of prana can help counteract these devastating effects of grief.

It is said that we receive prana in three ways: by Sun, Earth and Air. The primary and most constant way our bodies receive prana is through the breath. We also receive it through the food we eat and the water we drink. Higher concentrations of prana are found in fresh, pure foods. It is also in abundance in forests as trees take in, amplify and release prana as well as oxygen through photosynthesis. Prana levels in the atmosphere are high at mountain-tops and near bodies of water. There is abundant prana in nature. Grieving people can benefit immensely simply from going outside to consciously breathe and move.

Our bodies take in air which travels to our lungs. From the lungs, oxygen is transferred through the rest of annamaya kosha by means of the circulatory system. Prana does not follow this same delivery system. It enters and disperses immediately throughout the entire body. Because pranamaya kosha lies directly next to annamaya kosha, the physical body is directly impacted by and, in vital ways, is dependent upon pranamaya kosha. Likewise, pranamaya kosha is affected by annamaya kosha.

Prana is a force that can be directed, increased and decreased. It moves throughout the koshas via the *nadi* system. Nadi means "tube" or "channel" and comes from the Sanskrit root *nad*, meaning "flow." According to yogic sages, there are 72,000 nadi channels throughout the body. Our circulatory and nervous systems are gross nadis. The subtle nadi system is a similar system and in many ways corresponds to our physical nadis, but it cannot be seen by physical means.

Subtle and gross nadis function together and complement each other. When we experience trauma or illness, the subtle nadi system is affected and blocks can occur. Traumatic and prolonged grief can create blocks in the chakra system. The chakras are spinning vortexes of energy which affect the gross and the subtle bodies. While the chakras correspond with locations in the physical body, they do not reside in the physical space; they reside in the subtle body. The ancient Tantric seers, the first to map out the systems of the nadi channels and the chakras, perceived the main chakras as situated along a column of energy extending from the base of the spinal column to the top of the head, the *sushumna nadi*. The seven main spinning centers of energy are distributed upwardly along the column of sushumna. Chronic blockage or malfunction of any of these energy centers, which receive, assimilate and express our life energy, can result in physical, mental or emotional imbalance or illness.

Sustained blockages in the flow of prana and in the systems of the nadis can have profound effects. Trauma is frequently part of grief, as grief, with or without death, is almost always a part of trauma. Traumatic grief is multilayered and can have energetic, mental, emotional and physical affects that are long lasting and far reaching. Yoga practices, as well as other alternative therapies such as acupuncture, acupressure, and other kinds of energy work, can help with energetic blocks in pranamaya kosha and in the chakras.

Pranamaya kosha meditation

Sit comfortably, with the spine long and tall, but not stiff. Allow the hands to find a comfortable place in the lap or on the thighs. Tilt the chin slightly downward, lengthening the back of the neck. Slowly close the eyes to signal body and mind that you are now moving your focus and awareness from outside to inside. Imagine the eyeballs relaxing in their sockets, back and downward toward the heart center, allowing the focus to shift inward. Release the muscles of the jaw. Inhaling, roll the shoulders up and back, exhaling with a sigh, release them downward, creating space between the shoulders and the ears.

Bring your awareness to the breath. Notice as the breath moves in and out of the body. Notice whether you are breathing mostly through the mouth or through the nose. If you can, close the mouth and allow the breath to move through the nostrils.

Notice your unique pattern of breath. Let the breath be natural, unforced. Try to release any and all judgment of the breath. Notice the temperature of the air as it moves into the nostrils, down the trachea, into the lungs. Notice how the breath changes as it leaves the body. Notice the movement and the action of the physical body as the breath comes in and as it goes out. Notice how the body expands with each in breath and how it contracts on the out breath, gently rising and falling. Notice how the front of the body, the sides of the body and the back of the body expand. Notice how all of these contract. You do not have to do anything to change the breath, simply notice. Stay with this noticing of the breath for several cycles of inhalation and exhalation.

When you feel acquainted with the way the breath moves in and out of the body, slowly begin to expand the belly on the inhale, deepening the breath. Allow the front of the body and the sides of the body to expand further, creating more space for the prana-giving air that you are bringing in. Notice the movements of both breath and body as you deepen and expand with the inhalation and as you release and contract with the exhalation.

On the next inhalation, deepen the breath even further, allowing the belly to fill and then expand the ribs through the sides and back, filling the lower torso. Allow the exhalation to be slow and easy. Deepen the breath further on the next inhalation, expanding the belly, the ribcage, then allowing the chest and the collarbones to rise. Pause briefly. Allow the exhale to again be slow and easy, letting the collarbones and shoulders drop, the chest deflate, the ribs and then abdomen move inward, exhaling fully and completely. Continue breathing smoothly, practicing this deep three-part breath for a few more cycles.

Notice any changes you may experience in taking in this deep, nourishing, three-part breath. When you wish, return the breath to normal, maintaining the sense of expansion and ease with the breath. As you inhale, conceive of not only oxygen but of life-giving prana entering the lungs and moving throughout the body. Using your inner vision, send or direct prana into the feet and the toes. Breathe in, taking in prana with oxygen. Imagine the prana filling your lungs. With the energy of the exhalation, direct the prana where you want it to go in the body as CO_2 and toxins exit the body. Notice what you feel, sense or experience. How do you envision prana as it moves through the body? You might imagine it as cool flowing water, a golden presence, an invisible force; as waves, squiggles or spirals; as light, sparkling, twinkling, shining; as energy flowing, glowing, spreading. Perhaps it moves slowly, unfolding, undulating, expanding. Or it may move quickly, rushing, whooshing, zipping through the kosha, or immediately arriving as quickly as a thought itself, wherever in the kosha you ask or direct it to go. However it moves or does not move, notice any experience you may have—any sensation, thought, visual impression or feeling—without judgment or attachment to a specific outcome.

On the next inhalation, send prana to the hands, concentrating on the palms and then the fingertips. Do you sense, feel, or mentally envision any activity or change in perception? Direct the prana now to the soles of the feet. Notice any changes. Send prana now anywhere you feel you need support, soothing, healing, strengthening, expansion or attention of any kind. This may be an area of pain, tightness, injury, numbness or discomfort. It may be a place where you experience a sense of "stuckness," where the flow of energy may seem dampened or stopped. Maintain your attention on that area, inhaling and directing prana into the space. With each inhale, direct prana to that space of need.

With each exhale, notice further release of tension as well as any other sensations you may experience. Is there a sense of lightness, expansion, groundedness or melting? Is there numbness, heaviness, contraction or resistance? Without judgment simply notice what is there. What do you notice as the breath moves in and out? Direct the prana elsewhere if you wish, continuing this sending, directing and exploring of your ability to send and sense the energy, movement and effect of prana in the koshas. What else do you notice? What are your observations? Without judgment, simply notice how prana moves and behaves.

When you feel you have explored prana maya kosha as fully as you wish, open the eyes, bring the hands to the heart center in anjali mudra in gratitude to the life force within.

The third kosha—manomaya kosha

Manomaya kosha, the middle kosha, is our mental sheath, the thought body. It is closely associated with our nervous system and the place from which our thought waves, the vrittis, arise. Manomaya kosha is *manas*, the mind. It is our cognition, our thought-power. Neighboring pranamaya kosha, the breath and energy body, has a great impact on manomaya kosha and vice versa. When our minds are racing and we feel we cannot still our thoughts, focusing on and deepening the breath can slow the mind and calm the body. Our breath reflects our mental state. When our minds are overloaded, overwhelmed, anxious or worried, the breath may be ragged, shallow, uneasy, erratic. When our mind is at ease so is the breath.

Because pranamaya kosha lies between mind and body, it serves as a connection between the two. The body also reflects the state of the mind. Bodily symptoms such as tension, pain and anxiety can be exacerbated or relieved by our thoughts. The body carries and reflects the effects of trauma, pain, and stress. The breath can help ease some of the symptoms of pain and grief and, when expanded and free, can bring a sense of spaciousness for both body and mind.

Manomaya kosha is the center of management for many functions in the physical body including the senses as well as all cognitive function. An old and much used proverb says, "The mind is a wonderful servant but a terrible master." The mind does a great deal for us, working all day and most of the night, solving problems, remembering things, telling us what we think and what to do. It is in charge of interpreting, drawing conclusions and communicating about all the information it receives constantly through the senses; comparing and contrasting that from information stored within its extensive memory bank. It questions and it doubts. It wonders and it speculates. It pontificates and it preaches. It takes offense and puts up defenses.

Manomaya kosha is memory, emotion, ideas, feelings, imagination and originator of all kinds of thoughts about all of its own functions. It is very busy. It is frequently wrong about what it thinks, what it tells us and what it believes to be true. It is often highly reactive and sometimes gullible, but it usually means well. It is the sheath that gives us the mental power to operate daily in the world, to set goals and reach them, to believe that we have the power to achieve. It is changeable and malleable and when we learn to manage it, instead of the other way around, things tend to be much calmer inside and out. Manomaya kosha is the place where peace and chaos turn. It can be the most dangerous, the most painful, the most unpredictable, the most influential, the most potent and the most peaceful place for a person in grief.

In grief, the mind is powerfully affected. The way we think is changed. The content of our thoughts is altered. Particularly in early and traumatic grief, we forget things, we lose things, we are distracted and inattentive. Alternatively, we can be utterly focused on thoughts of our loved ones. We zone out, we draw blanks, we review, we scrutinize, we reject and we ask unanswerable questions. We may question the very foundation of our most deeply held beliefs. The way we saw the universe, other people, relationships, life itself, the way things are, can change drastically. We think about who we are now that this has happened to us, and try to decide how that makes sense based on who we were before grief came and what that will mean when we become whomever it is we will be in the future. We contemplate the strangeness of the loss of past interests and the inability to care about things that were once important. We wonder why other people continue to care about those things. We wonder what it all means. If it means anything. And how could this have happened? We have fears we never had before and we often find brave ways of talking ourselves out of them and of continuing on anyway. We ponder at the ways we are more fearless than ever before. We wonder why we are still here, how we will go on from this place and why we should bother trying. We worry, and at the same time do not care, what others think of us. We imagine our beloveds someplace or no place and wonder what it is really like where they are, if they are. We worry that we are crazy and that no one else could possibly understand. We feel deep connections with others who share this kind of pain and we are capable of understanding suffering, compassion and empathy in ways we never imagined before. We hate and we long to be alone with our thoughts. We have thoughts and feelings of guilt, regret, anger, unfairness, yearning. We search for relief, for answers, for signs of our loved ones' continued existence and involvement in our lives. We hope they are okay and safe and happy. We remember them and we miss them and we continue to love them and to long for them. All of this changes and then, in different ways, repeats. This is manomaya kosha in grief.

Manomaya kosha meditation

Sitting comfortably, allow your attention to simply be with the breath for a few cycles of in and out, inhaling and exhaling, noticing what you are feeling. When you are ready, bring the attention to the mind and to your thoughts. You do not have to change anything, you are simply noticing. What are you thinking about right now? Is your mind on the meditation, or are you thinking about what you need to do later? Whatever the mind is thinking is fine, you are simply noticing what is going on, the tone, the content, the happenings within the mind at this moment.

Our thoughts and feelings are always reflecting the three qualities of Universal energy, known as the *gunas*. These are *rajas*, *tamas* and *sattva*. If the mind exhibits rajas, there is a sense of being overstimulated, of racing, change, activity. The quality of tamas is sense of inaction, of being sluggish, sleepy or slow. The balance between the two is a sattvic state, the thoughts calm, peaceful, in harmony with breath and body. What kind of energy is present in the content of your thoughts at this moment? Is there worry, anxiety or judgment? Curiosity, interest or doubt? Calmness, distraction or ambivalence? You are simply noticing your thoughts. There is no right or wrong.

As you notice and observe the mind and its contents, begin to imagine the thought forms as clouds in the sky, moving through your field of awareness and then out. You do not have to become involved with the thoughts, you are simply noticing them. If you like, you can begin to label the thoughts as whatever they are: planning, thinking, worrying, daydreaming, fantasizing, questioning, remembering. Note the content, the quality, the tone of the thoughts. Watch them come and go and simply allow them to be what they are.

If the thoughts are overwhelming or too painful, you may choose to take a break from the mind and move back to pranamaya kosha, bringing the focus and awareness to the breath. When you feel ready, shift awareness back to the thoughts. Know that, if the contents of the mind are painful or frightening, you are safe in your space. It is the nature of the mind to shift and to change. It is the nature of the mind to find pain and remind us of it. You can know that you can experience painful thoughts, memories and feelings and you can be okay. You may choose to explore these thoughts, noticing and watching with curiosity and non-judgment, where they lead, what connections they form. Simply noticing and seeing the content of the mind at this time, on this day, watching the shifting sands of thought tumbling through the mind-stuff.

When you feel you have explored manomaya kosha as fully as you wish, open the eyes. Form anjali mudra at heart center or the brow in gratitude to your mind. Send a message of thanks for all the work the mind does for you each day, always doing the best it can to serve.

The fourth kosha—vijnanamaya kosha

Vijnanamaya kosha is the sheath of wisdom and intellect, of knowing and intuition. It is the place of discriminatory thinking that brings insight and deep understanding. It is the wisdom that lies beneath all the thinking and processing functions of the mind. It is the place of symbols and colors, of dreams and visions. It is your gut feeling and source of inspiration for all manner of creative acts. It is your place of perspicacity and discernment in all things. It is also a place of determination. When the mind is in doubt, it is *vijana*, or wisdom, that will finally come to a conclusive place of resolve.

We more regularly have clear access to vijnanamaya kosha when the first three koshas are functioning in a more *sattvic*, or harmonic, way. Because it rests next door to manas (mind) it can be greatly influenced by manomaya kosha. Our trust in our place of deep wisdom can be dampened and even damaged by messages we may receive from manomaya kosha.

In grief, we often lose sight of our own deep wisdom. Nothing seems to make sense, we don't trust our intuition. We no longer understand how the person we see in the mirror is the same person we understood to be "me" just days before grief and death visited our known reality. When the foundation of the universe shifts, when everything we thought was true is suddenly, clearly not true, it can be hard to trust in anything, especially ourselves and our own wisdom. The pain—physical, emotional, mental, spiritual—can be so deep and wide, we can be afraid to trust in anything again.

Sleep and dreams, a place where vijnanamaya kosha can speak to us, may be a comforting place of escape; they may bring visitations from our loved ones, which we long to trust but doubt to be real. Reality is what happens when we wake, we think. Dreams may also bring pain and fear, be full of trauma and rife with symbols of our grief. We have insidious and unwelcome thoughts about our other loved ones dying. When we say goodbye to our living loved ones as they walk out the door or as they drive away, it is nearly impossible to intuitively know that we will see them again, that things will ever really be okay.

Many bereaved speak of having "known" in some way their beloveds would die. Looking back, we sometimes recollect things that in retrospect seem to point to our intuitively having seen this coming—but there would have been no way to interpret such thoughts or feelings or notions at the time as such knowing. Some people report having had dreams or nightmares that depicted their loved ones in death, or dreams of other symbols that they could later relate to the manner of death or dying or surrounding circumstances that led to their beloved's death. Some recall the strange inability to imagine, envision or visualize their loved one past a certain point in the future.

These things then terrify us when we experience the very natural fear of the deaths of other loved ones. If our intuition seemingly foretold of one loved one's death, and we imagine or have dreams of living loved ones dying as a result of the trauma, how can we tell the difference between intuition and fear? Finding ways to manage and cope with this very real distress, now that we really, truly know that those we love are not protected from death, is work that can be best done in vijnanamaya kosha. The problem is that often we can feel very much separated from our wisdom body, which we may no longer believe we can trust.

To get to vijnanamaya kosha, we must first get past the mind. Moving beyond the mind's constant dialogue can be a challenge. Recent research from the University of Virginia showed that in 11 separate studies, most participants did not enjoy time alone with their thoughts with times varying from 5 to 15 minutes. In one study, many subjects preferred to administer a painful shock to themselves rather than be alone with no distractions. When the content of our thoughts is petrifying, bewildering and seemingly inescapable, this can begin to make sense. The difficulty though, is that grief ultimately cannot be escaped. Particularly in our Western culture, people in pain will do nearly anything to escape the agony and the accompanying thoughts, fears and imaginings that come with it. Drugs—prescribed or not—alcohol, work, exercise, hobbies, shopping, gambling, sex, risk-taking, adrenaline rushes of all kinds, anything to distract from the pain. We may succeed in distracting or numbing ourselves for a bit, but eventually, we are brought back to the grief, reminding us that it is part of us. Sometimes this happens when the next loss comes and more layers of grief are added on.

Vijnanamaya kosha is also the seat of the ego, *ahamkara*, literally the "I-maker." It is the voice of "I," "me" and "mine" that is useful for many things, including helping us survive. It is the ability to experience ourselves as separate beings. It is the "I" that makes each of us the very center of our own universe. Without it, we would be unable to experience ourselves as separate from others. In order to live as distinct beings in this world, we require the very thing we often seek to transcend. The goal of most spiritual paths is to experience the Oneness with All, to escape the feeling of separateness from God. But here is ahamkara, telling us we are separate. And in grief, we know, beyond any shadow of doubt, that we are separate. A widow grieving her husband of 47 years put it very succinctly when she said, "It's like you're...*set apart*...from everyone else. You're not like everybody else anymore."

A major function of vijnanamaya kosha is to help us function as separate beings in the physical world of dualities, going about our business, judging things, situations and people, in our own sphere of the world in a perfectly "normal" fashion. Then grief comes and ahamkara goes berserk. We are so separate that we feel concealed in a cover of isolation beyond anything we had ever previously imagined possible.

Ego is often thought of and discussed in negative terms, but ultimately it is a necessary function of consciousness. It cannot be eradicated. We can learn to use our wisdom to determine when ego is serving us or not serving us. Is it useful or is it destructive? Ego is necessary but can be a great source of pain when we identify too strongly with what it tells us about who we think we are. Comparing and deluding ourselves can be destructive forms of ego function. Yogic practices of meditation and self-inquiry (Jnana practices) can help us cultivate our witness and learn to be objective about what mind and ego tell us.

Vijnanamaya kosha meditation

Sitting comfortably, allow the spine to be long and tall, but not stiff. Let the muscles of the jaw relax, shoulders away from the ears, chest open. In this meditation, you may wish to form jnana mudra (see Figure 2.2, page 36). Rest the hands with the mudra formed, index fingers and thumbs touching, palms facing upward on the knees, the thighs or in the lap. Let the breath be smooth and even.

From here, allow the mind to use its power of imagination and visualization to move from manas into vijnanamaya kosha. Imagination is the place and space of the intuitive wisdom body. Allow your imagination to open. Visualize yourself in a place that is familiar and safe. This may be a room of your own home as it is now, or a place where you felt safe as a child. You may see yourself in a place that exists only in your imagination. This place can be any place you like as long as you feel safe, held and at ease.

Fully imagine this place and the space around you. Notice whether you are sitting or standing. What do you see around you? What are the colors, shapes, and objects surrounding you? What does it feel like? What are the textures, the temperature? Are you indoors or outdoors? What can you see? What details do you notice? Look around and see these things. What can you hear? As you look around the space, you notice a door. Regard the door. See it fully. What is it made of? Walk toward the door. Sense that this door leads to a safe space. Look down at the door handle. Notice what it looks like. Place your hand on it and open the door.

Find yourself now in a new place, look around. Notice what this new place is like. Are you indoors or outdoors? As before, take the time to notice the details of your surroundings. Do you recognize this place? You may or may not, but sense that you are completely safe here. What can you see, hear or feel in these new surroundings? As you take in the place, the colors, the space and its contents, your eyes come to rest on a nearby body of water. Notice the details of this body of water. Is it a brook or a stream? A river or a lake? A pond or an ocean? A fountain or a wading pool? What do you see?

Walk over to the water. Look down at your feet. If you are wearing shoes, remove them. Dip your foot into the water. Sit down at the edge of the water if you wish. Put both feet in the water. Notice how cool and refreshing, how calming and soothing, the waters feel against your skin. You may wish to put your hands in the water. You may wish to wash your hands, your arms or your face in the water. You may wish to drink the water. If you feel it's the right thing to do, immerse yourself in the water. Allow the water to embrace and hold you. Permit an encounter with these healing waters to occur. This water is part of your very being, giving access to your very own pool of wisdom. You can stay here or emerge from the water whenever you wish.

Looking up, you notice something new in the surroundings: an entry way in the distance. It may be a path, a gate, another doorway, a parting of the flora, a portal or some other kind of access. Notice a figure approaching. As the figure comes closer, you realize there is something very familiar about this figure. You know this figure intimately, even if you have never seen this figure before. This is the embodiment of your very own deeper wisdom. As the figure comes closer, you are able to see more clearly. Allow your wisdom guide to materialize fully. What do you notice? Is it human, animal, an elemental form or perhaps a version of your own self? Let it be what it is. Allow this embodied form of your wisdom to come closer. What does your wisdom look like as it reveals itself to you in this form at this time?

As you recognize your own wisdom, notice the feeling of love, safety, protection, well-being and deep intuitive knowing that comes with this recognition. Allow this encounter to unfold. Is there communication? If you wish, ask a question. Wait upon the answer. If you wish, reach out and touch your own wisdom body.

When you are ready to bring the encounter to an end for now, say goodbye in whatever way feels comfortable for you. Within your visualization, close your eyes. When you open them, the figure of your wisdom body has gone. Look around the environment once more. Notice whether anything has changed. Notice if your wisdom has left anything for you to remember this encounter. If so, pick up this souvenir and notice what it is. Put it in a safe place. If there is no souvenir, simply recall the feeling and the experience with your wisdom body. This is your gift. Bring your hands together at heart center and honor your own wisdom. Take a few deep breaths in gratitude.

Turn to see the door you came through to visit your sacred space. It is open, waiting for your return. Through it, you can see the safe space from which you came waiting for your return on the other side of the threshold. It is safe and inviting. Turn and walk back through the door into your safe space. Take a seat wherever you feel most comfortable. Take a deep breath, allowing your whole self to expand, exhale and, opening your eyes, find yourself back in this physical world.

Remember: Just because something may occur in imagination, or in the metaphysical, does not mean that it is not real. Write down as many details as possible of your experience with vijnanamaya kosha in your journal and revisit it later.

The fifth kosha—anandamaya kosha

Anandamaya kosha is the sheath of bliss. The experience of anandamaya kosha is the peace, joy and love that we experience outside of time, completely beyond the mind and its thoughts, emotions, feelings, comparisons or categorizations. *Ananda* means "bliss." The experiences of anandamaya kosha are those which are conscious but beyond description or measurement. It is the place of no words, when we cannot adequately describe our experience. It is the place of "no time" that comes when we lose ourselves in something that brings great peace or joy. It is always there, we carry it with us, but it is not reachable by will or by thinking, or through any power of the mind. It is something that is revealed only when we release any form of control or striving to reach it. It is the immeasurable, indescribable complete bliss of the present moment. It is the child completely lost in play, the musician fully immersed in the joy of the piece, the climber at the pinnacle of the mountain-top. It is losing ourselves in beauty, the merging of our being into the All without ever even noticing. Once we notice, then the moment is gone. This part of our selves when revealed is close to what we mean when we talk about Grace. Beyond anandamaya kosha, is the True Self, the soul. That part of us all which is never born and which never dies but exists eternally, where there is no separation, no duality, nothing and everything.

The bliss and joy of anandamaya kosha can be elusive, particularly in grief. We may feel we might never again experience joy or a sense of belonging or peacefulness ever again. This is not a true belief; it is what mind tells us, it is what grief tells us. Anandamaya kosha only waits for us to realize its existence. Even in the pain of grief.

Anandamaya kosha meditation

Allow the spine to be long and tall, but not stiff. Let the chest be lifted, as if there is an invisible thread pulling your sternum upward toward the sky. Let the shoulders roll up, back and down. Let them find space down and away from the ears. Tuck the chin slightly and allow the back of the neck to lengthen. Close your eyes.

Breathe in. Breathe out. Let the breath be easy and natural. Join the tips of the index fingers and thumbs on each hand to form jnana mudra (see Figure 2.2, page 36). Let the hands rest, palms facing up, on the knees, on the thighs or in the lap. Let the extended fingers and arms be relaxed, but ensure that the tips of index finger and thumb remain comfortably joined.

Bring your awareness to the place where the fingertips join the thumbs in jnana mudra. As you continue to hold this awareness, begin to notice that the longer you hold your awareness in this one-pointed space, the tips of the fingers begin to feel less and less like the tips of your fingers. Let the sensation move from one of pressure to that of expansion, of melting, of tingling. Allow your experience of this sensation to expand, to become larger, as if from that point of joining, all particles of your being become rarefied, less dense, expanding into the space around you.

Allow this sense of expansion to move into one of dissolving. Allow the dissolution of the tips of the fingers and thumbs. Allow the dissolution of the hands in their entirety. Dissolve the wrists, the arms and the shoulders. Dissolve the space where the hands were touching the legs, then the legs themselves, thighs, calves, ankles, feet and toes, expanding, dissolving. Dissolve the chest, back, neck, head and face. Allow the heaviness and solidity of your entire being to dissipate, all molecules floating, expanding and dissolving as if into a vast sea of tranquility. When your entire being is dissolved, allow yourself to rest in this state. Feel no separation from the space surrounding you. Know that you are completely free in this limitless space of openness. Know that all stress, tension, anxiety, pain, fear and exhaustion have also dissolved into this vastness.

As you rest here, gently and without judgment, observe any thoughts, ideas, notions, insights or feelings that may arise. Allow those to be seen and then also dissolved into the selfsame space that is you. Know that any and every bit of consciousness can arise and be dissolved and accepted fully into this Oneness of which you are part and which is part of you, and which is you. Nothing is too heavy, too much or too big to be embraced and accommodated. There is no judgment, no separation. All is One. Resting, floating, merging, opening, expanding, being. Here is the blissful all-encompassing state of anandamaya kosha in which you can rest freely and fully and which is always here for you, in you, and of you.

When you are ready to end this meditation, send your consciousness outward and begin to gather together your molecules. Bring each molecule, each particle, each cell, back together; allow them to re-form, taking the shape of you once more. Bring your awareness to the space where your index fingers and thumbs are joined in jnana mudra. Press the fingers together, noticing the change in the pressure. Bring your awareness to the sensation of pressure and the tactile sensation against the backs of your hands as they rest on your legs or in your lap. Bring awareness to the sense of pressure as you sit, where your thighs, feet, and legs are touching the chair, the floor, the cushion. Bring your awareness to the space in which your body is now resting. Note the temperature of the room, any sounds you can detect, the feel of your clothing against your skin. Come into this present moment, here and now, as you fully inhabit your physical body once more. Bring awareness to your breath and allow it to deepen. Let the breath out with a deep sigh if you wish. When you are ready, gently open the eyes.

Working with energy

Our subtle energy system is housed within pranamaya kosha. Our energy body reacts and interacts with the other koshas. The centers of our energy are the chakras. In Sanskrit, the word chakra means "wheel" or "circle," and also "to turn." There are many of these energy centers throughout the body, but the major chakras are situated along the sushumna nadi, the major energetic pathway which corresponds with the spinal cord in annamaya kosha, the physical body. The seven major chakras interact with annamaya kosha, as well as with manomaya and vijnanamaya koshas, the mental and wisdom bodies. While the health and functioning of the chakra system influences our ability to enter into awareness and direct experience of anandamaya kosha, it does not directly impact the bliss body, as it is always there, always in bliss, regardless of our perceptions or experiences in the other four sheaths.

The system of the chakras is fundamental to understanding the movement and flow of energy in the koshas, and the chakras play a major part in all systems of holistic and alternative healing methods. The positions of the major chakras correspond to physical places in the physical body (Table 4.1). Under assault from the extreme stress of grief and bereavement, our physical and energetic systems are greatly affected. The chakras and their functions are vital to our general health and well-being. Typically we hear of chakras being "open" or "closed," but those terms do not accurately reflect the complexity of the dynamic energy centers. Any chakra can be balanced and sattvic, with energy moving harmonically in and out. Chakras may be in active states, energies moving in a healthy equilibrium of input and output. They may also function in more passive states, meaning the chakra is at rest. Any of these three states, active, balanced or passive, can mean the chakra is functioning in a healthy manner.

Table 4.1 The major chakras and their correspondences

Chakra	Symbol	Color	Sound	Element	Physical body	Body sense	Endocrine gland
1st Base/Root Muladhara		Red	LAM Musical note C	Earth	Perineum	Smell	Testes/ Ovaries
2nd Sacral Svadisthana		Orange	VAM Musical note D	Water	♀ Sacrum/ Cervix ♂ Sacrum/ Top of pelvis	Taste	Adrenals
3rd Solar plexus Manipura		Yellow	RAM Musical note E	Fire	Just above navel	Sight	Pancreas
4th Heart Anahata		Green/Pink	YAM Musical note F	Air	Center of the chest on the sternum	Touch	Thymus
5th Throat Vishuddha		Turquoise	HAM Musical note G	Ether/ Space	Base of the throat	Hearing	Thyroid
6th Brow/ Third eye Ajna		Deep blue	OM Musical note A	Spirit	Center of the brow	Extra- sensory perception	Pituitary/ Pineal
7th Crown Sahasrara		Violet/Gold White	OM Musical note B	Spirit	Top of the head	All senses known and unknown	Pineal and all of endocrine system

Chakras may be overactive, reflecting a *rajasic* quality, meaning the energetic center may need calming or balancing. They may have blockages, be underactive, or *tamasic*, requiring stimulation. Any of these states can occur when the energetic system is seeking balance within the physical or mental bodies. Tamasic or rajasic states may result when adverse conditions such as illness, stress, shock, trauma or grief affect the energy body.

Learning to be familiar with energy and increasing your ability to recognize, follow and shift prana throughout your koshas can help you move toward a more sattvic state of harmony, even in grief. Tantra gives us tools that can help us better tolerate, detect and create energetic shifts in the koshas, as well as to increase, decrease, move and balance energies within our subtle and gross bodies and throughout the chakra system. This affects and creates changes in our physical, mental and emotional states. In grief, we so often feel that we have no control over what is happening to us, within or without, but with some knowledge of the energetic system and some basic tantric tools, we can learn to better manage some of the intolerable energetic and emotional states of grief.

In yoga, the goal is always to seek, create and move toward the more sattvic state, a state of harmony, a balanced state of body, mind and prana. When we are grieving, nothing seems or feels harmonious. Our energetic state in grief can range from beyond lethargic, an indescribably heavy sadness, like a lead blanket weighing us down—tamas—to the manic, pacing, caged animal feeling many are familiar with in grief—rajas. In the grip of either of these states, grieving people can find it difficult to imagine ever feeling in harmony with anything ever again. The tools of Tantra can help us move toward center, where we can come closer and closer to state of sattvic harmony, within and without.

Yoni mudra

Mudras have long been used in tantric practices. The mudra's energetic seal directs and promotes prana within the koshas and encourages a sattvic state. *Yoni* is the Sanskrit for both "vulva" and for "origin." Mukunda Stiles, in his book *Tantra Yoga Secrets* (2011), encourages the use of yoni mudra before every tantric practice, as well as before sleep and upon waking to encourage the tantrika to connect with prana and deepen the ability to recognize and detect pranic energy and movement.

Yoni mudra is a powerful mudra that helps to create a connection between the sacral and heart chakras, our energetic centers of creativity and of love. Yoni mudra also provides sacred connection with Goddess energy, increasing our sense of connection with the Source. Yoni mudra is particularly useful in balancing the energies of the first three chakras—root, sacral and solar plexus—and can be beneficial in helping to ease energetic trauma to these areas.

To practice yoni mudra, place the palms of the hands downward, flat on the lower abdomen, with the thumbs aligned straight across, and the index fingers touching, creating a downward pointing triangle or delta shape (Figure 4.2).

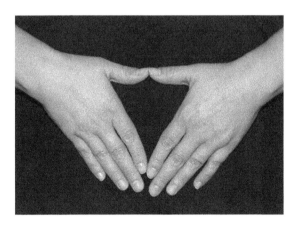

Figure 4.2 Yoni mudra.

If the fingers overlay, allow the left hand to be on top of the right. You can practice yoni mudra seated or lying down. Initially, simply begin to notice the natural pattern of your breath. As you inhale, notice where the body naturally expands. You may wish to use the three-part breath, filling the abdomen, the rib cage and then the chest. Then exhaling in the opposite way, allowing the chest to deflate, the rib cage to move inward and the abdomen

144 | *Yoga for Grief and Loss*

to pull in toward the spine. Continue this slow, deep three-part breath. If you become dizzy or lightheaded, return the breath to normal.

As you breathe in and out, begin to become aware of the energy of your body, notice whether it feels low and heavy, or high and restless. Notice whether you sense more energy in certain areas than others. Notice whether the energy seems to flow in different places in the body, or if it seems stuck or stagnant in any particular area. Everyone's experience of energy is different. If your consciousness is drawn to particular areas of the body, it may be that these areas are holding a high concentration of prana, or that these are areas where the prana is blocked or stagnant. Explore those areas. See if you can notice the exact spot where your attention is drawn and focus your attention on that space.

You may perceive sensations of tingling, vibration, swirling or pulsating. If you are a more visual person, you may envision colors, patterns or images associated with your pranic energy. Thoughts or feelings may arise that are associated with the movement of your prana, or you may experience kinesthetic or physical aspects of energy movement and location, such as muscle twitches, shudders, heat, chills or goose bumps on the skin. Remember to allow what is to be.

In the practice of yoni mudra—however you notice and experience your energy—begin directing the energy—tamasic or rajasic, low or high—into the space created by your hands as they hold yoni mudra. Ask the energy to move to this space; visualize the energy flowing toward the space, like water moving toward its source; envision the space of the mudra as an energetic magnet, drawing the energy into the space. Imagine the energy here expanding and growing. If you wish, visualize prana as light, or as a silver or gold ball, glowing at your center.

Allow the breath to be deep and slow, directing energy into the sacred space of the yoni mudra until you begin to feel more centered. Once you feel that you have completed your exercise, release the mudra. Press your hands onto your pelvic bones. Imagine anchoring or storing this energy in the pelvic area for future needs. In grief, this practice can help to create a sense of groundedness and of connection. It can be a tool for self-care to be used at any time you may need centering or grounding. It is also helpful for relieving anxiety and to help calm the mind.

Honoring the elements and ourselves

Tantric practices encourage the fullest experience of the world around us. For the tantrika, the full use and appreciation of all our senses is spiritual practice. In the yogic and Tantric philosophy and teachings, each of the five elements of nature—Earth, Air, Fire, Water and Ether—corresponds with one of our five physical senses, as well as with a chakra center. Our energy is part of creation and is dynamic even when we don't recognize it as such. In times of grief and loss, our energy may not feel very active or flowing, but we are always in sync with creation. Creation is never static and includes within it contraction as well as expansion as part of the evolutionary process. In times of grief, loss, pain and trauma, we may be in a state of contraction more often than expansion. This is normal. It should be expected. Contraction, moving inward, protecting and closing off is a normal response to what, in traumatic grief, is an overwhelmingly abnormal situation. Expansion is the next normal response, when opening comes again.

Like all of nature, because we are part of nature, we move in cycles through contraction and expansion. This movement is physically represented in an asana and in the breath. In grief and trauma, we see the same movement. Going inward, moving out again—contracting, expanding. Doing this mindfully, and sometimes purposefully, helps us move toward a more sattvic and therefore a more comfortable state.

Nature strives toward homeostasis, and as part of nature, so do we. We humans do not like change—and certainly not chaos—but change inevitably happens, and grief is one of the most chaotic times of life that we will ever experience. Small events can be shattering, such as hearing a certain song, seeing seemingly loving families spending time together, stumbling across your beloved's old tennis shoes. In a state of stability these things—a song, the sight of a loving family, a pair of beat-up Nikes—would not create a problem, but in the chaotic state of grief, we can be completely undone by the smallest things that suddenly expand into the biggest things.

Rituals both large and small can help us better manage the chaos of grief. In many ways, all of Tantra is about ritual. Tantra's essence is rooted in approaching life wholly, fully, abundantly, in this world, in these bodies, in having the purely human and fully spiritual experiences that we do and understanding them all as holy. Rituals, both sacred and secular, help to bring order, aid us in transitions and help us to understand complex feelings. Through observing our own senses, acknowledging how we are feeling and purposefully using the tools of ritual to safely come into the present moment with our grief, with our love, and with whatever else the moment holds, we can find ways of moving through each moment and into the next. In grief, this can be an essential practice.

In Tantra, sacred rituals are known as *puja*, pronounced "poo-jah," a word meaning the act of worship. The purpose of worship is to cultivate awareness of our own higher consciousness and of our connection with the Divine and with our own True Selves. When we are living in alignment with our True or Higher Selves we are also living in alignment with the Divine Force of creation. The ritual puja shared here is an adaptation from Mukunda Stiles' puja to the five elements found in his book *Tantra Yoga Secrets* (2011). It is meant to deepen our connection with Mother Earth through our own sensory experiences.

To practice this puja, you will need to prepare your own personal altar space. Suggestions and guidance for creating your own altar space are shared in the Bhakti chapter (see Figures 3.1–3.3, pages 69-74).

Gather the items you will need before you begin. You will need items to represent each of the elements—Earth, Water, Fire, Air and Ether—which also correspond with our five physical senses of smell, taste, sight, touch and hearing respectively. Each of these corresponds also with a chakra center. The correspondences are these:

- The Earth element corresponds with the sense of smell and with the root chakra, Muladhara.

- The Water element corresponds with the sense of taste and with the second chakra, the sacral chakra, Svadisthana.

- The Fire element corresponds with the sense of sight, the third chakra, the solar plexus chakra, Manipura.

- The Air element corresponds with the sense of touch, the fourth chakra, the heart chakra, Anahata.

- The element of Ether or Space, corresponds with the sense of hearing and the fifth chakra, the throat chakra, Vishuddha.

- The other two chakras, Ajna the third eye and Sahasrara, the crown chakra, are beyond the five elements and the physical senses. If you wish to acknowledge and represent them on your altar, a good choice is to have crystals or stones present which correspond to those chakras. Good examples of very affordable stones are lapis lazuli or iolite for the third eye chakra and clear quartz or amethyst for the crown.

See also Table 4.1, The major chakras and their correspondences (page 141) as a reference.

Spend some time thinking about the objects you might use and begin to gather them. Be creative; think about the correspondences of the elements, the senses and the chakras in choosing the ritual items that appeal to you. Preparing for a ritual—deciding on and gathering the items you choose to represent the elements, your senses, and figuring out how you will use them—is the true beginning of the ritual. As we imagine, think, plan and choose, we begin to bring our minds into a calmer state as well as begin to gather energy for the ritual itself.

After your altar space is arranged, begin your ritual. You may begin by chanting Om, saying a prayer, singing a song, striking a chime or engaging in any other method to symbolize moving from ordinary space and time into sacred space and time. Next, make and place each of the objects as offerings on your altar. Pick up each item you have chosen to represent each sense. Wave it slowly in a clockwise circle toward the center of the altar. Bow to

Spirit as you place each back on the altar. Moving in order from the Earth element (root chakra), begin by making and placing an offering that is pleasing to the sense of smell. Next, honor the Water element, by offering a food with a delicious taste (sacral chakra), then light a candle for Fire and the sense of sight (solar plexus chakra). Next, make your offering to the Air element and the sense of touch (heart chakra). Finally, make an offering of your symbol for Ether and the sense of hearing (throat chakra). If the offering is your voice, sing or chant your offering and then bow to Spirit.

Make each offering a second time, spending time with each of the senses. This time, touch each corresponding chakra space on your body before making the offering of the object. This creates an energetic connection between the physical body and the energy body by way of the senses. This is a Tantric practice known as *nyasa*, which means "placing." Nyasa places divine and elemental energy into our being while it creates the energetic connection between annamaya and pranamaya koshas, the physical and energy bodies. As you practice nyasa, touching each chakra space, and then engage the senses with each elemental offering, be aware and mindful of the way each offering stimulates and engages each of the senses.

Be fully present as you contemplate the object which represents and honors your sense of smell and the Earth element. Holding the object in the right hand, offer it once again to the altar. With the left hand, touch your body as close as possible to the root chakra space. Contemplate the object. Notice its shape, its weight, its color. Deeply inhale the scent and let the aroma permeate your olfactory space. Imagine the energy of that fragrance blooming first in the space of the root chakra and then upward as it moves through the chakras and the koshas. Where do you sense the energy? What sensations do you notice? Savor the flow of the energy of the fragrance. Place it on the altar.

Take up the offering representing Water and the sense of taste with your right hand. Wave the offering in a circle again toward the center of the altar. As you hold the object with your right hand, touch your body with your left in the sacral chakra space, at the lower abdomen. As you taste of the food or drink, allow it also to please your other senses as you mindfully contemplate its color and texture. As you place it in your mouth, hold it there for a moment and savor it. Become aware of how that particular food or drink came to you. Was it grown in the Earth, nourished by sun and rain, harvested by human hands? Was it transported across miles or grown close to home? Does it contain more than one ingredient? Has it been altered by heat or flame? Notice what happens in your mouth, how your tongue and teeth hold the food or drink item. Can you taste more than one ingredient? As you chew and swallow, notice the movements of your jaw, tongue and throat. Feel it move through your body, eventually to become part of annamaya kosha.

Next, offer your lit candle once more. While holding it in your right hand, touch the space of the solar plexus chakra with your left, about two fingers above the belly button. Place the candle on the altar. Pass your hand by or hold it safely near the flame. Feel its warmth and heat. Gaze at the flame, notice how it dances, how it moves. Notice how the colors of the flame shift and change. Be fully present with the flame as it glows and warms the space of your altar.

Offer next your object representing the sense of touch and the Air element. Again, holding the object in your right hand, touch the area of the heart chakra with your left hand. Contemplate its texture. Is it bumpy, smooth, soft or coarse? Notice its color, its shape, as you feel and touch, tracing the edges of the object, its center, all of its sides. Note how it takes up space. Is it solid all the way through? Does it hold spaces where air could move through? Touch it gently with your fingers. Let the tips of the fingers glide across the surface gently. Massage and explore the object with a deeper pressure. How does this change your experience? Close your eyes. How does this change your experience of the touch?

Finally, present and experience your chosen offering to the Ether element and your sense of hearing. Touch the base of your throat with the left hand, connecting with the throat chakra. If music is the offering, be fully present. Allow your ears to drink in the sound. Close your eyes to more fully engage with sound. Allow the energy of the music to move through your koshas. Move your body to the music if you wish. If you offer your voice in song, chant or prayer, close your eyes and allow the vibrations of your voice to move throughout your koshas. Know that the sonic vibrations of this sound offering will continue to travel through space, carrying the energy of your worship through the universe.

To close your ritual, bring your hands to anjali mudra, say a special prayer or closing chant, ring a chime or any other signal of ending that you choose. Put out the flame and thank the Elements and Spirit.

You may wish to make this puja to the elements a daily or weekly practice to continue to honor and connect with the Divine within yourself and within the Earth. Particularly for those in deep grief and for those who have experienced all kinds of trauma, this ritual can help to create a sense of safety and connection.

Creating your own rituals

Creating your own personal rituals allows you to access grief in a safe and structured way. A ritual can be as elaborate as a public memorial service or as small as a quiet moment alone with your loved one's picture. You may even already engage in your own rituals without realizing they are rituals. Here are some suggestions:

- Light a candle at certain special times of the day or week to remind you of your loved one.

- Create a memory scrapbook and fill it with photographs, letters, postcards, notes or other significant memorabilia from your life together.

- Spend time listening to your loved one's favorite music.

- Watch his or her favorite movie.

- Make a playlist or a special CD of music that reminds you of your loved one.

- Plant a tree or flowers in your loved one's memory.

- Make a donation to a charity that your loved one supported.

- Visit your loved one's burial site.

- Carry something special that reminds you of your loved one. Hold it when you need to.

- Create a work of art in your loved one's memory.

- Cook a special meal in honor of your loved one.

Some people engage in smaller or spontaneous rituals on a regular basis such as some of those listed above. You may do the similar kinds of things or you might choose to create more structured rituals. You may decide to create a special ritual to occur only once, or you might decide to hold your ritual on a regular basis—daily, weekly, monthly, or on special days like birthdays, anniversaries, holidays or other special times.

More formal rituals tend to follow a basic structure. They include preparation—such as arranging the altar or other sacred space where you plan to hold your ritual—an opening, a middle, and a closing. Clearly marking the beginning and the ending of rituals helps us move into a different frame of mind, into sacred space, and then signals that it is time to shift our consciousness back to an ordinary mode of being at the closing.

Here are some suggestions for openings and closings of rituals:

- Light a candle or some incense.

- Read or say aloud an inspirational verse, poem or prayer.

- Sing, chant or play a particular piece of music.

- Ring a chime or a bell.

After the opening, take a few deep breaths to center yourself. Remember that all feelings are okay within your ritual space and within your grief. A ritual is your space and time to express grief and love in whatever ways you choose and need to do so. Whatever happens in between the opening and closing of the ritual is completely up to you. You can have an activity planned, such as working on a memory book, writing a letter to your loved one, planting a tree or flowers—the possibilities are unlimited. Or you might have nothing planned. After the opening, you might wish to simply sit quietly for as long as you need to, listen to music, spend time crying, look through photos of your loved one, meditate, pray, read some healing literature or a sacred text. It is okay to do whatever comes to you in the moment.

Sometimes you may feel the need to communicate something to your loved one. The sacred, safe space of a ritual is an ideal place to do this. When you need to communicate, you may choose to speak aloud, meditate on your thoughts silently, or write your thoughts in a letter. You might include the burning or burying of the letter that you write within the ritual.

You may simply feel the need to release energy in your ritual space. Yell, scream, or cry as much as you need to. If you're working with feelings of anger in your grief, keep pillows nearby that you can hit, punch or throw. Tearing and ripping paper or stomping cardboard boxes can also help release anger. You may wish to include some movement, dance or vocal expression such as singing, chanting or yelling. You might want to beat on a drum or play some other instrument to release energy and emotion through sound.

You can conduct rituals alone or with others. Your ritual could be an ideal time to share your grief with friends and family members grieving the same loss. If you share your ritual, you may wish to ask each person to relate something about your lost loved one—a memory, story or thought. They may wish to participate in your ritual activity such as chanting, drumming or letter writing. You might ask them each to bring something to read or share as part of the ritual.

You can conduct grief rituals for as long and as often as you need or want to. You may find that your need to engage in ritual for grief will wane. Everyday rituals, such as carrying your loved one's photograph, or wearing a particular sentimental piece of jewelry or sleeping with an item of clothing, may also shift over time. You may feel the need to hold more structured rituals only on special days such as birthdays or anniversaries or not at all. This is all okay. Change is natural. Everything in nature, including us, changes. Rituals help us move from chaos and pain to wholeness and stability. They are always there when we need them.

Suggestions to cultivate a Tantra practice

- Practice yoni mudra and follow the energy in the body regularly.

- Spend time with Nature as often as possible.

- Talk to plants and animals. Imagine that they hear you. Imagine what they might say back to you.

- Walk barefoot or lie on the Earth.

- Plant a garden, a tree, flowers. When you tend it, engage with it as a conscious being.

- Acknowledge the Feminine Divine in ways that are natural for you.

- Explore the Goddess in art and history.

- Spend some time—an hour or a day—with the intent of offering every action as ritual, as sacred acts, given to the Universe.

- Practice ritual on a regular basis.

- Regularly create and engage in delightful sensory experiences.

- Spend time focusing on each of your chakras, devoting a week or a day to exploring aspects of each.

- Go to the ocean, a lake, a river, a creek or some other body of water and listen to its song.

Chapter 5

Karma Yoga

The Path of Action

The word Karma comes from the Sanskrit root *kri*, meaning "to do." All action is Karma. Every breath we take, every movement, every choice, every decision, large or small. It is the work that we do, the play we engage in, the rituals we practice, the mistakes we make, the love we give and take. It is also the sum, the total, and the resulting effects of all our past actions. This does not mean punishment as many mistakenly believe. Karma is not the Universe's mechanism for "payback" or retribution. It is the Universe's mechanism for the balancing of energies.

Karma yoga is service to others with the release of attachment to the fruits of the outcome. Karma yoga helps us to shape our own Karma and find freedom from the isolation of grief, the pain of every day existence and, ultimately, the wheel of Karma, into the spiritual freedom of our souls, known as *moksha*. Karma yoga is doing for others. It is work done that helps others and humankind. It is practicing service and kindness.

As yogic science indicated centuries ago, modern science is showing through a growing body of research that Karma yoga actions, performing altruistic acts to benefit others, have long-term physical and mental health benefits. A study on the effects of volunteerism on depression, conducted by Musick and Wilson in 2003, found that mental health benefits of volunteerism included increased feelings of happiness, an increased sense of well-being and a reduction in symptoms of depression. The Corporation for National and Community Service's 2007 review of research on volunteerism and service revealed the presence of increased "positive feelings, referred to as 'helper's high,' increased trust in others, and increased social and political participation" as well as "a greater sense of purpose" for those who gave of themselves in service to others (p.3). In a 2003 study, Schwartz, Meisenhelder, Ma and Reed investigated whether giving help was a more important predictor of better reported mental health than receiving help. They found that, of the nearly 2000 individuals in their study, helping others was associated with higher levels of good mental health, and rated above and beyond perceived benefits of receiving help.

Teachers instruct that in performing Karma yoga we are to offer our actions to God, to the Universe or to humanity. The ultimate goal is to allow our work to be transformed into purely selfless service to others. In grief, as in life, this is much easier said than done. However, when actions come from a place of love, whether the act is selfless, self-motivated or driven by the desire for our beloveds to be remembered and known, the love itself can direct the outcome. When love drives the action, our personal motivation ceases to matter as much. Swami Vivekenanda taught in a series of weekly lectures given freely in his New York apartment in 1896:

> We have to begin from the beginning, to take up works as they come to us and slowly make ourselves more unselfish every day. We must do the work and find out the motive, the power that prompts us; and, almost without exception, in the first years we shall find that our motives are always selfish. But gradually this selfishness will melt by persistence, till at last will come the time when we shall be able to do really unselfish work. (Vivekenanda, 2013, p.4.)

Swami's words seem an almost perfect description of the unfolding of Karma yoga in grief. In my own experience, and in my conversations with all grieving people who have delved into service and volunteerism in memory of their beloved dead, in the beginning, the work, the devotion, the dedication, the acts of service, are almost exclusively about our personal need to ensure that others remember our beloveds, as well as our own vital need to continue to feel connected to our beloveds through physical acts. We need to know that someone else knows they existed, that their names, their faces, their lives are not forgotten. We need reassurance that their presence—as well as the absence of their presence—meant, means and will continue to mean something. Finding and making meaning is significant, and necessary to the integration of our experiences of grief and loss. Over time, and through the work itself, the acts become less about us and our own needs and, also, if you can imagine such a thing, less about our beloveds themselves. The work becomes more and more about the work itself; about extending the love within outward. It is a reflection of the light of our beloveds and of our love for them onto the world. It becomes more about how the work itself gradually makes us more compassionate, more open, more empathetic, more loving and more giving. Service and kindness are love and compassion turned outward—empathy in action. These are gifts from our beloveds that we can hold close and from which we can gain strength.

Karmic balance

The concept of Karma is comparable to Newton's third law of motion: For every action, there is an equal and opposite reaction. We take a breath, we give it back in a different form. Every action results in a consequence or an effect. This includes non-action. To choose not to act has an effect. Understanding this can make us aware that every action we take, and each choice we make to refrain from action, has consequence. Consequence includes a return of energy. Equally, events and circumstances, and their effects upon us, occur due to a previously corresponding cause. When something happens, something else must have happened prior to create the effect that we find ourselves experiencing in each present moment.

In terms of Universal reciprocity, actions and consequences do not have assigned values that equate to our limited human understanding of the Universe, God and Its workings, nor to our dualistic and uniquely human conceptions of "good" or "bad." Actions and choices are reflected and returned with comparable energetic qualities—some of which we may understand and some which we may not. Some perhaps, with our limited ability to comprehend the entirety of the Universe and all Its workings, we cannot understand. This is reflected in Biblical teachings such as Galatians 6:7, "That which a man soweth, he shall also reap," and Ephesians 6:8, "Whatsoever good thing each man doeth, this shall he receive again."

Other religions, spiritual and cultural traditions have similar Karmic concepts. Many Wiccans and pagans hold to a tenet termed the "Law of Three," which states that whatever energies one sends out into the Universe will be returned to us threefold. This may be interpreted by some as good will reap good, but ultimately the Law of Three, as well as Karmic law, doesn't always have an immediate impact that can readily be measured. If I donate three dollars to charity, I won't necessarily get nine dollars back later; this could be the case, but more accurately the Law means that my energies are returned to me threefold from a metaphysical perspective. If my actions create what I might see as good, at some point, I may receive in a conscious way what I might call good, but it is far more likely that I will never know the true outcome or return of my actions.

Outcome, as well as return, also depends on intent. Many things impact the kind of return we receive for our actions, the Karma that we create. The type of energetic space in which the action was taken, whether I am emotionally attached to the outcome of my actions, what I hope or do not hope to receive as a result, and whether the action was done out of love, selflessness or a desire to be in alignment with my True Self and the higher good all impact the type of Karmic return I will later reap. The Law of Three, as well as the law of Karma, means that our actions and choices affect us in three potential ways, on the levels of mind, body and soul—mentally, physically and spiritually/energetically. This is the threefold return, which is not necessarily measurable or visible.

Other ancient and tribal people held to similar Karmic rules which extended also to the planet. In the Celtic imagination and belief system, the land was not simply matter, but truly alive. They lived their lives based on the held knowledge that the actions of each individual impacted the entire world around them—family, friend, neighbor, animal, Earth. The Celts' concept of ethical responsibility had to do with the deep understanding that we each are part of the landscape of the Earth and also part of each other. To harm one's neighbor or the land was to harm one's own self, body, mind and spirit. Many Native American traditions have similar concepts of ethical causality and Divine justice echoing these same principles.

Karmic laws of Universal balance and return have nothing to do with punishment. There are systems of thought that indicate, and many people believe, that if we do bad things, we get bad things. We will be punished. When something terrible happens, including the deaths of those we love, many grieving people agonize over why they are being punished, why their loved one was punished. Ideas of magical thinking can run rampant—if I only think good things I will receive good things; if I think bad things, bad things will happen. I must have done something bad. While it is the case that our current realities are partly determined by our thoughts, we decide lots of things—where we are going to go today, what we will eat for lunch, what color to paint our walls. But just because we want something badly, or do not want it, does not mean that reality will come to pass. Grief is not the fault of the griever.

In the same vein, there are those who believe that, if only we have enough faith, then what we pray for will come to pass. Following that if/then construct, if we do not have enough faith, then we will not be rewarded. These kinds of feelings can have a huge impact on our experiences in grief, trauma, illness and adversity. When friends, family, society and popular culture send the message that somehow your lack of faith, your lack of positive thinking, your lack of belief has created this painful circumstance, it feeds the notion, secretly held by many, that this is true. We are doing it wrong and we are responsible. Grieving people are frequently sent this message, overtly and tacitly.

To believe that what we think brings us good or brings us bad and that we are the authors of not only success or failure, but health, life, death and even tragedy is to become caught up in magical thinking. This can create a great deal of anxiety as well as unnecessary guilt and shame. So many of the great spiritual leaders are right in saying that it is not our circumstances themselves that are problematic, it is what we think about them that create our distress. The grieving Hamlet said, "there is nothing either good or bad, but thinking makes it so." Our thoughts are powerful and have a great deal to do with how we see our world and everything in it. This is not the same as our thoughts creating our literal reality. We can and do have impact and effect on the world around us—our reality—but there are also so very many circumstances where reality is completely out of our hands.

The three Karmas

There are three types of Karma. *Sanchita*, which means in Sanskrit "heaped together," is often likened to a personal storehouse of Karma. It includes all that we see, do and experience over every lifetime from the very moment our souls come into being. We bring our Sanchita Karma with us with into every incarnation. All the impressions that form and accrue through the events of every lifetime come with us until all our Karma is completed or burned away through spiritual practices. Annamaya kosha, the physical body, is the only sheath that is shed at death. All the other koshas continue on, carrying the imprints and impressions of Sanchita which are reborn with us each lifetime. Sanchita Karma is also the accumulation of all action and Karmic work that we have done; impressions and the collected fruits of our work from life to life.

With each birth, we come into life with certain Karma that has become ripe and which will be expressed in that lifetime. This Karma is known as *Prarabdha*. In Sanskrit, the word means "action unleashed" or "commenced." These are inevitable events that will happen to us in this life and over which we have no control. This is destiny. That may sound daunting, to some it may sound silly. But in Karmic Law, it is a certainty that there are things that will happen in each and every lifetime which cannot be changed or avoided.

Thought of in another way, the concept can bring a certain sense of comfort or relief. If we have no control over certain things that will unfold, we can sometimes find a way of releasing resistance; we are more able to integrate the experience into our being. We can most easily do this when we have a sattvic, balanced nature. We must also understand that our Karma is influenced by and entwined with the Karma of others. Every person we meet, to greater and lesser degrees, has an influence on our Karma and how it unfolds, as we have influence on theirs. This means that what happens to those we love is their Karma as well as ours. This includes the responses of all involved, which is part of why we all need to care for one another.

While Prarabdha is inevitable, all other Karma is in constant flux. We always have the ability to choose our responses and shape future Karma, including future Prarabdha Karma, based on our responses. If we do our best to ensure that our actions and our reactions come from a place of love, where we, and our intentions, are as closely aligned as possible to our True Nature and our Highest Selves, to Love, we can feel as close to assured as possible that the outcome will be the most appropriate and the most needed for any future circumstances.

Often we can look back and see what appears in hindsight to be an unfolding of occurrences having paved the way to major events in our lives—including sometimes the deaths of those we love. We may be able to look back and see how our lives seemed to prepare us in many ways for major Karmic events in our lives. Not all Prarabdha Karma is undesirable. Some may be very desirable or beneficial. Often these are also things which we can look back upon and wonder at how unfolding events seemed to conspire and urge the Prarabdha Karma into its inevitable fruition. No matter whether the things that happen to us are painful and aversive, or profitable and advantageous, each of us has the task of how we will respond and react to Prarabdha, and this creates future Karma.

That future Karma is the third kind of Karma created and shaped in each moment of our present lifetime. Known as *Agami*, it is Karma yet to come. Also known as *Kriyamana*, the word comes from the Sanskrit for "to do," *kriya*, and *manas*, mind. It is the Karma which we set in motion with our present consciousness and actions. It is the Karma which we are creating now and which will eventually ripen into Prarabdha Karma in future incarnations. Kriyamana is that Karma over which we have the most control and with which we can mold our futures. An image often used by teachers to describe Karma is that of an archer. The quiver holding the arrows is Sanchita Karma, the storehouse. The arrows in the quiver which the archer must carry are her Prarabdha Karma, inevitable Karma. The quiver and the arrows it holds are given to her at birth. As she reaches into the quiver, selects an arrow, draws her bow, aims and releases, she is exacting personal control over her current Karma. This is Kriyamana. Once the arrow is let go however, she is no longer in control. This becomes future Prarabdha Karma. We can do our best to have good aim, but at the final moment, we must simply trust and, as much as possible, let go of expectations along with our arrows. We are always carrying our quiver and its arrows and we are constantly selecting and firing new Kriyamana Karma off into our futures which become our inevitable Prarabdha Karma. In order to live the most peaceful and balanced life, we must learn to release our attachment to the outcome of our efforts. When we do this work with consciousness and self-awareness, this is Karma Yoga.

Karmic conditioning

Karma is also the force that conditions and shapes our souls from lifetime to lifetime. It has a large part in the formation of individual personality and shapes our character from life to life. As pleasure and pain, happiness and sadness, pass before us and imprint their effects upon us, we take in that which we learn from each event and we act according to the way our minds and hearts direct us. Much of this inner direction is based on the impressions we carry with us from life to life; from birth to death to rebirth. In yoga these impressions, held in the subconscious mind, are called *samskaras*. In each life, we acquire more and more samskaras which continue to impact our actions and choices. Each action and choice leaves its mark upon us. In the West, a close approximation to this is what we call temperament. The more self-aware we become, the more influence we have over the interplay of our Karmic temperament with our circumstances and our impact on the outcome of occurrences.

In terms of Karma, the more free from delusion and illusion our consciousness, the more insight we have into our own motivations. The more we move from a place of love and selflessness, the more we can form new samskaras and shape our own Karma, in this and in future lifetimes. In the Hindu, Buddhist and Jainist religions, the ultimate goal is to break the cycle of Karma; to be released from the cycle of birth, death and rebirth. The Sanskrit term for this freedom is *moksha*.

I have certainly known many bereaved who have wished to be released from the agony grief can bring. Living with circumstances which have created the kind of indescribable pain that traumatic grief can bring is one of the most difficult tasks imaginable. To wish to be free of the pain that life can bring is an understandable desire. To know that we have a part in shaping our own destinies, even when we feel powerless, can help us withstand and move through the pain of grief and trauma. This is not to say that to understand Karma, or even to shape Karma, is to be released from the suffering of grief in the now, or grief yet to come, but rather that through our choices we can have some control over our current circumstances and potentially, if you choose to believe it, over future circumstances, both in this lifetime and beyond.

Having a better understanding of Karma can help us to be aware that each action has effect. There are those who may say that based on Karmic law we are helpless in the face of tragedy, grief or pain; that since whatever is happening is a result of some past action or event over which we now have no control, there is nothing we can do and are therefore powerless—Prarabdha Karma is unfolding no matter what. While it is true that there is nothing we can do to change the past, the present, and our actions in the present, are constantly shaping the next moment and then the next. The future eventually becomes the present and then the unalterable past. We can participate in and shape our own destinies, and our futures, by being aware and mindful of ourselves, our emotions, our motivations, and making choices that reflect our highest and truest selves. The truth which is revealed in all branches of yoga—and of all true spiritual paths—is that our True Self is Love. When we move forward in love from all places and spaces, the Karma that we create, and that which is returned to us, can be only for the Highest Good—that which is for the greatest evolution, growth, nurturance and love for our own True Self as well as for the whole of humanity and the universal collective One. This is the way we can become released from Karmic bondage— patterns of behavior and their resulting energetic returns that cause us pain.

Guilt and shame in grief

Karma in grief can be a difficult concept to wrap our minds around or to even try to understand. But even the attempt to do so can help to provide some relief and widen the path that can move us closer toward a deepening peace with the workings of the Universe and our part in it. We may never understand why our beloveds had to die in tragic, painful ways, or before they had the chance to live long, full lives. Questioning—why her, why him, why us, why this way, why not someone else, why violence, why pain or suffering?—can create more anxiety, additional pain and self-condemnation on top of existing grief, even though it is completely natural to do so. Reviewing events, ruminating over what think we did wrong, what we could have or should have done differently that may have avoided the tragedy or resulted in some different outcome are extremely common among people who have experienced the death of a beloved as well as those who experience trauma and loss due to other events such as violent crime, abuse, even natural disasters.

Sometimes finding a peaceful place within for the questions themselves can be a saving grace. The resounding "WHY?" rarely has any forthcoming good answer. Allowing the questions to simply be without seeking an answer is a freedom in itself. Practicing a meditation where you can simply observe the questions and imagine them taking a shape or form and resting in an inner space can be helpful.

Meditation and visualization

Finding a place for the questions

Come to a comfortable seated or lying position. Bring your awareness into the present moment. Bring your attention to whatever is supporting your body. Notice what is beneath your feet, your legs, against your back. Notice where your body is touching this support and where it is not. Notice the temperature of the air in the room. Notice the feel of the air on your skin. Notice the sounds you can hear in the space outside where you are and the sounds within. As much as possible, without judgment, begin to notice how you are feeling. Briefly scan your body from the soles of your feet to the top of your head and back down again. Notice the places in your body where you may be holding tension. Without trying to change anything, send prana by way of your breath into those tense or painful spaces in the body. Allow those spaces in the body to soften and relax a bit further.

Begin to notice your feelings and emotions. Bring your awareness to the places in your body where these emotions and feelings are being held or stored. Without feeling that you need to change these emotions or feelings, send prana via your breath into those spaces. Notice whether the feelings shift, if the emotions alter in any way. Note whether they seem to move or grow or stay the same. Allow whatever you are feeling to be, for this moment, just as it is.

Begin to bring your awareness to your breath. Close your eyes if you are comfortable doing so. Notice how the breath is moving in and out of the body. Simply stay with your breath for a few inhalations and exhalations. Notice the way the body moves with the breath, rising and falling, expanding, contracting.

When you are ready, bring your awareness to the question or questions that your mind seems to focus on the most. Allow the questions to rise. If you begin to cry, remember that this is okay. If you do not cry, this is okay too. If at any time you experience increased tension, pain or any kind of distress in the body, breathe into the spaces and places where you experience this and see if you can soften those places. Know that whether or not the questions can be answered is unimportant in this present moment. For now, simply allow the questions themselves to rise and to be. Notice where in your body you feel the power of the questions resonate the most. Notice the tone and the energy of the questions. If you can, imagine the shape, the color, the landscape, the texture or the terrain of the questions. Continuing to notice the places the questions are felt most intensely in the body, and without having the need to do anything about them, allows the questions simply to be.

Shifting perspective in your mind's eye, imagine now that you are looking at yourself from the outside. See yourself sitting or lying just as you are, in this space. See your face, your body, your clothing. Note the position of your hands, the placement of your feet and legs. See how your belly rises and falls gently with each breath. From your current vantage point, send calming and loving energy toward yourself as you rest peacefully in this space.

Direct your gaze now to the place or places on your body where the questions resonate most strongly. Imagine that you can observe the questions beginning to leave your body. Perhaps you might see them appear within a thought balloon above your head or to your side. Perhaps they seep out like mist, emerging as figures, shapes, objects, animals or something else entirely. Notice the shapes or forms they take when they are outside your body. Know that the questions are not harmful. The questions are simply removed inert from your mind and body. They have no power. They simply are. Simply witness the questions.

Imagine now a box, a chest, a closet or some other storage space of your own conception; a space where you can place the questions and allow them to simply be. If you really need to look at them or examine them at any future time, you can always come back to them. See the questions in their visualized form become small enough to place into the storage area and imagine moving them with the power of your mind into that space. Know that the questions are comfortable and safe here in this space. You can shut the lid and close the door and leave them there for safekeeping as long as you wish, and you can go back and look at them or think about them anytime you want. Notice now whether you can detect any difference in your body, your emotions, or feelings. Notice what thoughts are going through your mind. Simply noticing all of these things without judgment and without the need to strive for anything to be other than what is, right now in this moment in your body, your feelings, or your mind. When you are ready, take a deep, full breath, release it, and open your eyes.

Sometimes our questioning has also to do with personal responsibility. *Why didn't I know? What if I had done something differently? What if this (or that) had (or hadn't) happened?* Reviewing and perseverating on *should have, could have,* and *if only* is completely normal and very common, but not especially useful, particularly when we hold on to or become immersed in that thinking. It adds pain on top of pain. All too often bereaved and grieving people feel punished and personally responsible for their own pain, heartbreak, misfortune and grief. While Karma does bring focus specifically to our actions—to causality as well as personal responsibility—the role of intent in Karmic effect cannot be underestimated. The intent of our actions, whatever they are, shapes the energetic effect as well as the return.

Guilt in grief has to do with blaming ourselves for what went wrong, for the horrific outcome that occurred. Blame implies intent to do harm. Most of us whose beloveds have died can look at the situation and agree that no, of course we did not, and would never wish or intend harm to our beloveds. No action was ever intended to cause harm, pain, suffering or death. Still, the guilt may be there.

Grief and guilt can become painfully entwined. And upon guilt is often layered shame. I have known and spoken with so many people who struggle with guilt and shame following the death of a beloved. The granddaughter who feels guilt and shame for not visiting her elderly grandmother who suffered with Alzheimer's because it was just too painful. The wife who laments asking her husband to run by the store on the way home when the detour resulted in a fatal accident. The many mothers, having suffered miscarriage and stillbirth, tortured by wondering whether what they ate or drank, or didn't eat or drink, or if that burst of cleaning and nesting, or going for that run, or lifting heavy things, working too much, overdoing it, wondering if they were ready for a baby, resenting being pregnant, caused miscarriage or early labor. They struggle also with the deep sense of shame that their own bodies failed them and failed their babies. Even when there was nothing she can think of that she did wrong, shouldn't she just have known somehow that her baby was in distress instead of going about her business like everything was fine? How could she have not known her baby was dead in her womb? So many people hear similar refrains in their minds: Shouldn't I have been able to protect? Shouldn't I have been able to change things? Couldn't I have kept it from happening? Often these kinds of thoughts don't even make rational sense. Yet the guilt is there. And the shame is there. The guilt says, "I did something wrong," and the shame says, "I am wrong." Wrong in how I grieve, how I mothered, how I cared for my beloved, how I performed my duties as a spouse, friend, lover, mother, father, sibling, grandchild.

In many cases, the guilt and the shame are supported by others—actual people as well as societal judgments and constructs that suggest implicitly or explicitly that they should have known, they should have done better or different. Others who believe that they themselves would never have taken their eyes from their nine-year-old child as he swam, those who believe they would never tell a suicidal ex-boyfriend they would not take his calls, those who believe they would never attempt to move a heavy piece of furniture with their baby in the house. Every grieving person doesn't experience this necessarily overtly, but that element, no matter how small, is present.

It is helpful to try to come to an understanding that Karma and all Karmic results are never a form of punishment. From a Karmic perspective, any punishment, real or imagined, is self-inflicted. When we identify strongly with guilt and shame, these feelings in themselves can become punishing. This is also not to say that you *should not* feel guilty or that you *should not* feel shame. In my experience telling someone to not feel guilty is completely useless. And "should" or "shouldn't" are not helpful. Practice in self-reflection and forgiveness can help us to understand what we may gain from inflicting this kind of punishment on ourselves and can help us find ways to dissolve it. This does not mean taking responsibility where we have no responsibility, but rather seeing our responsibility with open hearts and eyes. Rationally and intellectually we may be able to say that we have nothing to feel guilt or shame about, but emotionally these intellectual talking-tos don't always work.

You may wish to return to the loving-kindness meditation in the Bhakti chapter as a regular practice to help soften and open your heart toward yourself. The following is another meditation in softening and working toward releasing feelings of guilt and shame.

─────── Journaling and meditation exercise ───────
Softening and releasing guilt and shame

With a notebook and pen by your side, find a comfortable seated position. Allow your spine to be long and tall, but not stiff. Take a few deep breaths to relax the body and begin to come fully into the present moment. Look around. Take notice of your space and where you are in this moment. Notice any smells or sounds in the space. Notice the temperature of the air, notice the feeling of the seat, the cushion, or the ground beneath you. Notice where you may be holding tension or where you have any discomfort. Make any adjustments to bring yourself into a comfortable, seated position.

Set an intention to simply be with your feelings with as little judgment and as much self-compassion as possible. Bring your hands to anjali mudra (Figure 2.1 on page 30) and say, "For this moment, I release all fear. For this moment, I release all anxiety. For this moment, I release all judgment. For this moment and in this work, I intend to practice as much love and compassion toward myself as possible. This is my intention." Breathe in that intent. Repeat the intention if you feel you need to.

Bring your awareness to your breath. Simply breathe normally and calmly for several breaths. When you are ready, bring your attention to any feelings of guilt or shame that you may be carrying. Notice whether you have a sense of "I did wrong." This is guilt. Notice any sense of "I am wrong." This is shame. Notice what you are telling yourself about the guilt or about the shame. Notice the messages your mind is telling you. In this moment, if you can, cultivate a witnessing presence toward these thoughts, simply noticing what the messages are. Witness these as if you are hearing them from someone else, a person you love and care for. If you wish, stop for a moment and write down the thoughts. You might want to write something like:

> "The messages I am telling myself right now about guilt and
> shame are _____
>
> _____."

Returning your focus inward, bring your attention again to the feelings. Notice where you feel the feelings in your body. With curiosity and openness, bring your awareness to the space in your body where the guilt or shame is currently residing. You may hold these feelings in more than one place. Notice how they feel in that space of your body. What energies do the feelings carry? Are they still or do they seem to move? Do they feel dense, sharp, insubstantial, stealthy? Hot, cold, somewhere in between? Do they seem hard or soft, tight or loose? Are there any shapes or images that come to mind when you explore the feelings? Write down your impressions of the feelings.

"The feeling of guilt/shame in my body is like _____

_____.

Its shape is _____.

Its energy is _____.

It feels like _____.

It reminds me of_____."

Going inward again, move back into the space where you hold the guilt or the shame. Explore the space again, gently, as a witness, with curiosity and openness. In your mind or aloud, say what the guilt is. You may wish to write this down.

"I feel guilty because _____

_____"

Bringing your focus inward once more, allow this thought and statement, "I release this judgment of guilt."

In your mind or aloud, say what the shame is about. You may wish to write it down.

"I feel shame because _____

_____"

Bringing the focus inward again, allow this thought and statement, "I release this judgment of shame." Breathe for a moment and say: "I release these feelings and these judgments of guilt and shame." It might help to write the release down on paper.

As you say and write these things, imagine the feelings leaving the body, dissipating in the air, leaving through a window, disappearing into the sky or being absorbed into the Earth. In your mind, or aloud, to the sky or the Earth, a deity of your choice, or even your beloved dead: "Thank you for helping me to release these feelings." Breathe gently into the space where you once held these feelings. As you breathe into the space, imagine filling the space with pure love. If you wrote the release statements on paper, you may wish to burn the paper or tear it into small pieces and bury them under a tree. Thank the fire, the sky or the Earth for taking these feelings. You may wish to write down your thoughts and feelings about this experience. Know that you can repeat this exercise anytime you feel the need.

In grief, it can be hard to think beyond our current experience. Sometimes we can feel pain for others who are also in grief. Often we may grieve on behalf of our beloved dead the lives they will no longer experience. In general though, deep grief is extremely narcissistic, meaning that in grief our feelings are overwhelmingly about ourselves and our own personal and immediate experiences within that pain. This is not a bad thing, this is just what it is and it is often exactly what and how it needs to be. The contracting and moving inward must be about our own personal inner experience. These feelings are our own unfolding Karma. It may be a helpful exercise to think too about the Karma of your beloved dead.

Recognizing the death of your beloved and the surrounding events as part of their own Karmic path can in some ways help us to see that the Karma we are living is not ours alone. There are many things that are completely out of our control, even within the framework of our responsibility for our own Karma. Whatever yours or your beloved's Karma, they are most assuredly entwined. What part is yours and what is your beloved's can be difficult to separate. But there are certainly aspects that are separate. Our Karma is ours alone and also entwined with the Karma of others. As the famed comedienne Lily Tomlin once said, "We're all alone in this together."

Once we have departed our bodies, the Karma we have accrued across lifetimes will continue to unfold in the next lifetime and in the next. In some cases, your beloved's Karma may have been completed in this life. The Karma of our beloveds in this lifetime can no longer be altered, and may be complete, but ours, as long as we are living, is not yet done for this life. While there is no good or bad in Karmic law, and we may even at some point decide that the greater good is unfolding even with our pain, we can certainly perceive our lives without our beloveds as wholly undesirable and unfair. We don't ever have to like it. That doesn't mean you can't also experience love, compassion and forgiveness. Part of moving through grief and working with Karma is acknowledging what you are experiencing in this present moment as much as possible without judgment and from a place of love.

The universal forces of Karma help us to keep learning, progressing, growing and evolving throughout each lifetime. Even if you do not believe in multiple lifetimes or reincarnation, this can still hold true—we can always be growing. Ultimately, Karma assists us in the realization that our actions have effects which can be immediate and which reach far beyond that which we can see or realize in this current moment and perhaps even within this current lifetime. Through Karma our souls' paths cross and intersect and the resulting effects of even the smallest interactions can have effect in ways that we may never comprehend in life. Some souls meet time and time again to help further and ultimately complete the work of each of the souls involved. Some may meet only once but with great impact. Our interactions with each other impact the Karma of the whole. Karma teaches us that we can take responsibility for our actions and helps us come to a place where we can release expectations and attachment to the outcome of fruits of our actions. Karma also teaches that we can come to a place of peace with what we experience in our lifetime. This can seem very difficult to grasp or believe, especially when we are in pain. Practicing compassion toward ourselves, asking for forgiveness from ourselves, as well as from our loved ones and others, can help us to release judgment and feelings of condemnation and conditions which we may place on ourselves or others.

Love, forgiveness and gratitude: Ho'oponopono meditation

The Hawaiian practice and concept of Ho'oponopono means to *make things right*. This includes making things right with ourselves, with others, and with the Universe. It is a balancing and includes the righting of wrongs. In a sense, it is a reshaping of Karma we are currently living and also shapes our future Karma. When done with an attitude of pure love, this practice can help heal many injuries done to ourselves or others, as well as those that others have done to us. Forgiveness does not involve anyone but ourselves.

Ho'oponopono is also an ancient spiritual cleansing and clearing ritual. It reaches the self on all levels: mental, emotional, physical and energetic. Ho'oponopono removes stress and fear, anger and anxiety. The process assists us in being in touch with our inner Divinity and helps us to have a working relationship with that Divine inner nature. When we are in touch with who we truly are, all matters can be set right within. Ho'oponopono allows for any blemish on our conception of our true wholeness to be erased. Any erroneous thought or action can be cleansed and cleared, and all energies balanced. The process works with our ancestors, including our beloved dead, with living people, animals and with the planet as an organism. When we experience deep love, true forgiveness, genuine gratitude and make amends with ourselves, we can experience this energy from outside ourselves as well.

To practice: Find a comfortable space. You may wish to practice this in front of your altar or other sacred space. Take a few cleansing breaths, allow your heart and mind to be open.

Begin to chant or sing:

Ho'oponopono, ho'oponopono, ho'oponopono, ho'oponopono,
Ho'oponopono, ho'oponopono, ho'oponopono, ho'oponopono.

I am Sorry. I Love You. Please Forgive Me. Thank You.
I am Sorry. I Love You. Please Forgive Me. Thank You.

Repeat until you feel complete with your practice.

Our beloveds have already forgiven us. God and the Universe have forgiven us. Before we even ask, this is true. Forgiving and loving ourselves can help us to return to our natural state of wholeness.

Your service to others

Following a personal Karma yoga path may seem simple to some, while others may have no idea where to begin. Karma yoga, service to others, can be as simple as spontaneously helping someone carry groceries, holding a door, letting other drivers out in traffic. You may choose to donate to your loved one's favorite charity or volunteer for an organization that your beloved would support, or one which helps those who are dealing with grief, illness or another cause that is dear to your heart. You may wish to think about your personal talents, skills and abilities and how you may donate your time and talent to others. Think about how much energy you have to realistically devote to a project and always take care of yourself. In early grief, you may not be able to do anything for anyone else. You may be barely able to do anything for yourself. Later, when you feel stronger, you may wish to purposefully act to create your own Karma yoga service in the world, for yourself, and for your beloved.

Community Karma yoga

There are moments when entire communities affected by grief and loss can come together to perform services to assist both themselves and the community as a whole. These kinds of community Karma yoga acts are evident in community vigils and community-based groups that form to help improve living conditions, reduce crime and provide resources in urban, suburban and rural settings.

It is important to note, however, that community responses to grief, loss and tragedy can sometimes occur counter to the needs of the family and individuals directly impacted by the painful events. Many family members who have lost loved ones in highly publicized tragedies, such as school shootings, like those at Columbine, Virginia Tech and Sandy Hook, as well as individual cases which receive copious amounts of media attention, often experience anger, pain and resentment that their personal pain is seemingly taken over by community members and organizations. While vigils, funds, non-profits and other Karma yoga projects meant to both lessen the pain for the community and help others are noble and usually well intentioned, no action for the community or organizational purposes should ever be done without the consideration, and permission, of those who are grieving the immediate and visceral loss of their beloved ones. When this occurs without concern or thought for these most vulnerable, not only can more pain be created for these individuals, but the long-term and farther-reaching effects of the Karma yoga can be tainted. What we do to one we do to all.

The kindness project

Dr. Joanne Cacciatore, psychotherapist, teacher and researcher at Arizona State University, is also a bereaved mother and founder of the MISS Foundation, an international, volunteer-based non-profit organization supporting families grieving the death of a child. On July 27, 1994, Joanne's daughter Cheyenne was stillborn. Joanne speaks of that day as the worst of her life. At Christmastime that year, Joanne was, like so many bereaved and grieving parents, devastated at the prospect of a holiday without her youngest daughter. She decided the money that she would have spent for Cheyenne's gifts would be spent on underprivileged children anonymously. That act brought the closest thing to joy, as well as a deep feeling of connection with her daughter, that she could have imagined on that painful holiday. Joanne writes in her interactive workbook, *Selah: An Invitation Toward Fully Inhabited Grief* (2013),

> This sparked a pattern of very random, anonymous acts of generosity which I discovered were more healing to me than beneficial for the recipient. I created a 'kindness card' which could accompany the good deed and began telling others about it. The idea quickly spread through the bereaved parent community and on July 27, 2011, the day we would declare International Kindness Project Day, more than 10,000 people around the world united on a single day to use free Kindness Project cards to commit random acts of anonymous kindness in memory of a beloved child or parent or spouse or friend who died. While these good deeds do not eradicate grief, nor should they do so, they do provide a means through which the mourner can redirect painful emotions into feelings of love and compassion and hope. (p.59)

Here are some kindness ideas that may help to inspire your own personal Karma yoga actions.

- Make a batch of cookies and share them with neighbors or friends. You might want to do this anonymously.

- Tape quarters to a vending machine for the next person to use.

- Make a card or draw a picture for someone you love.

- Create small care packages in sealable bags including lip balm, sunscreen, water, a dollar or two, snacks. Give them out when you see homeless or people asking for money.

- Pay the bill for the next person in line at the drive-through or a toll booth.

- Make a piece of art and give it away.

- Leave extra big tips for servers in restaurants.

- Think of someone who has helped you in your grief, or at another time in life, and write them a letter thanking them, letting them know how they made a difference.

- Offer someone who is rushed or who has more items to go ahead of you at the store.

- Offer a sincere compliment to someone.

- Give a gift to someone for no reason.

- Ask how someone else you know who is going through a difficult time how they are really doing—and listen to their story.

- Place sticky notes with messages of kindness on public bathroom mirrors, in random places—in shops, tucked into grocery store flower bouquets, around your workplace, on the bus, in a taxi. They might say things that you would like to read yourself. *You are beautiful. I love you. You are not alone. You can do this.*

- Make a note of local charities and non-profits whose missions reflect your or your beloved's values and learn more about volunteering. When you feel ready, call.

- Donate dog or cat food to your local animal shelter.

- Make copies of your favorite photos of family and friends send them the people in them.

- With sidewalk chalk, draw pictures or write inspirational quotes or messages in public places.

- Send a copy of a book that you love or that you have found helpful to someone else.

- Send a care package to a soldier far from home.

- Leave a book with a note for the person who finds it in a café or airport or other public place.

- Pick up trash when you see it.

- Plant a tree in your loved one's memory. Plant several trees.

- Create a memorial garden and lovingly care for the plants and flowers.

- If you read something that is helpful or inspirational on a blog or social media, leave a comment letting that person know that their words or posting helped you.

- Each day, ask the Universe for opportunities to serve and to be kind to others. Take them.

Other suggestions to cultivate a Karma yoga practice

- Set aside a day of the week for Karma yoga immersion. Dedicate every single act that you do for the day to the Highest Good of all beings including yourself. In your meditations, include this prayer: "For this entire day, let me be totally selfless. Let every action I do come from a place of service and of love. I release all attachment to the outcome of my service to the world."

- Before doing anything, ask yourself, "What is my motivation? How will what I am about to do help others?"

- In any interaction, ask yourself whether you are contributing to or contaminating the situation.

- Practice loving-kindness meditation on a regular basis.

- At the beginning of each day, begin with a ritual of asking that each of your actions be a blessing to others. Let this be a touchstone throughout your day.

Chapter 6

Raja Yoga

The Path of Royalty

lso known as the Royal Path, Raja yoga is an integral practice which includes aspects of each of the other branches of yoga. The Sanskrit root *raj* means "to rule." The word *raja* itself means ruler, one who rules; a king or a queen. The path of Raja is meant to help us become just, fair and compassionate rulers of our own selves and our own minds. It is meant to help us understand ourselves more clearly and to be the best selves we can be—fully illumined, conscious, harmonious, integrated humans living peaceful and useful lives, regardless of our circumstances, places or stations in life. Raja yoga is also known as the path of the mind and the path of meditation. Mastery of the mind, rather than the mind being master of you, and the bliss that can follow, is the ultimate goal and, as Patanjali teaches, an inevitable outcome when our practice is firmly diligent, sincere and ongoing (sutra 1:14).

The Yoga Sutras of Patanjali, introduced in the chapter on Jnana Yoga, is the classical text used in the teaching of Raja yoga. Through the system of Raja yoga, Patanjali offers specific and useful tools to assist the bereaved as we travel the long and painful road of grief. For some, that road is life-long and as the *Sutras* tell us over and over, it is all practice. All of life, which includes all of grief, is yoga. Patanjali's gift is that his writings only point the way. He gives us the threads—the literal meaning of the word *sutra*—and with those threads allows us the opportunity to bring our own direct knowledge and experience to the process and product of the weaving, which belongs only to us.

Patanjali tells us, in sutra 1.14, that our "practice becomes firmly grounded when well attended to for a long time, without break, and in all earnestness" (p.20). One might read that sutra and feel discouraged or overwhelmed. Perhaps you might think something like, "I will never be a yogi! If I have to practice without break I'll never achieve it!" But think of it this way: all of life is practice. You get no break from life as long as you are living it. Patanjali doesn't say how long the time is, he simply says "for a long time." Without break doesn't mean that you'll be holding a specific asana or posture, or chanting the same mantra, or sitting in meditation for hours upon hours or day after day without stopping; it means that we practice being as fully aware as possible of our minds, our thoughts, our actions, of how we see, think, feel and do, and how our ways of thinking and doing impact our lives as well as the lives of others.

This kind of practice is possible whether we are on the yoga mat, cleaning the house, attending a retreat, going to the grocery store, sitting in meditation, going to work, staying home, hiding, laughing, crying, avoiding, breathing. Life is the practice. It is absolutely possible to "for a long time and without break" attend to being self-aware, conscious and as awake as possible.

The last part, "in all earnestness," is, to me, the easiest. Earnestness means with sincerity, with resoluteness, with a firm desire to have a strong groundedness in the practice of yoga and of a wholehearted and balanced life. This crucial sutra reminds me of the Zen Buddhist concept of *shoshin*, or beginner's mind: having an attitude of openness, a willingness to experience, without judgment or preconception, whatever is happening in the moment, in your practice, in your journey. No matter our experience, our education or background, we each are beginners daily, in life and in grief. Each day upon waking we can experience a new beginning, even in each moment and in each experience we can cultivate and experience new beginnings. Our practice is our lives. Our grief is part of the practice—it is a very, very difficult part of the practice. What you can do, at any point in the practice, with awareness, in all earnestness is yoga. Your practice is your life and your life is your practice.

Ashtanga—the eight-limbed path

Raja yoga is also known as Ashtanga yoga. The word Ashtanga itself means "eight-limbed." These eight limbs of yoga are the core of the teachings of Patanjali. Practiced together, the eight limbs create balance and harmony. The limbs focus on the overall goal of soothing the mind's restlessness, attending to the body and managing life so that one can function in health, peace and harmony.

No limb is more important than any other and they are to be practiced as a whole. Like trees, each human has several limbs—legs, arms, trunk. Our lives produce fruit and the health of the fruit depends on the health of the tree and of the person, mentally, physically and spiritually. The limbs of Ashtanga support all aspects of a whole person. Each limb is part of a holistic whole which, when practiced for a long time and without break, like the other branches of yoga, brings that same wholeness to the individual and reveals our eternal connection to the Divine.

Briefly, the eight limbs are these:

- Yamas—five conditions of behavior, things we should refrain from doing in order to live a harmonious and ethical life. They are *Ahimsa* (non-violence), *Satya* (truthfulness), *Asteya* (non-stealing), *Brahmacharya* (restraint) and *Aparigraha* (non-greed).

- Niyamas—five qualities to be practiced and cultivated for self-discipline and inner strength leading to a healthy body, mind, and spirit. They are *Saucha* (purity), *Santosha* (contentment), *Tapas* (discipline, pain, heat), *Svadhyaya* (self-study) and *Ishvara pranidhana* (surrender).

- Asana—the physical postures.

- Pranayama—yogic breathing practices to control and direct the life force.

- Pratyahara—withdrawal of the senses from the external, directing of the consciousness inward.

- Dharana—contemplation and concentration.

- Dhyana—meditation.

- Samadhi—experience of pure consciousness and bliss, the Oneness of Yoga.

In grief, as with so many things, the limbs of Patanjali's Ashtanga yoga may take on different hue. The typical way that Raja and the eight limbs are taught, explained or understood may not seem to work or to be as relevant when we are in grief. However, the limbs of Ashtanga can be very helpful for those in grief. In grief, through loss and in the aftermath of trauma, Raja yoga is about self-care, awareness and exploration of our own experience as well as a guide to functioning in the moment and in the long term as we attempt to integrate the experiences and results of grief in our lives. Above all, the practice is about becoming and remaining fully conscious, in life, in pain and in grief.

A sutra worthy of discussion before moving into the eight limbs is one that can offer hope and guidance toward increasing our ability to grow, to learn and to care for ourselves in our grief. Sutra 2:33, "*Vitarka badhane pratipaksha bhavanam,*" says this: "When disturbed by negative thoughts, opposite/positive ones should be thought of. This is pratipaksha bhavana." This sounds very simplistic and, in a way, it is.

Early in grief, most of us can no more change our thoughts than we can change the weather. The idea may seem preposterous and even offensive. But just as water can steadily and slowly carve a canyon into a mountain of stone, we can, over time and with practice, replace traumatic, painful and destructive patterns of thinking with those of a more peaceful, harmonious and sattvic nature.

The first step is being aware of damaging thoughts. Watching the thoughts, noticing how often negative or harmful thoughts come, seeing how they affect our feelings, mood and peace of mind, questioning whether they are true, introducing something positive, and then paying attention to whether or not, or how often we can change the thinking is a worthwhile practice. It may be helpful to remember that Patanjali doesn't just say to have "positive" thoughts; *opposite* thoughts are encouraged. So if the thought is one of fear, think of the opposite of fear. Depending on you, this might mean peace, trust, courage, love, any number of things. At the right time in your journey, the practice of pratipaksha bhavana can be a powerful tool. It is one that is made more precise and effective with the accompanying practices of mindfulness and meditation. The exercise below may be a good practice to begin the practice of pratipaksha bhavana and also to help quell anxiety and repetitive, harmful thoughts.

Experiential practice

Pratipaksha bhavana meditative breath

When you can isolate negative or harmful thoughts, distill them to one or two descriptive words. Once this is done, spend some time thinking of what the opposite concept or word is. Choose an opposite that you truly believe you can cultivate to increase the effectiveness of the exercise.

Close your eyes, lengthen the spine to free the energy flow, and inhale slowly and deeply, allowing the abdomen to expand. With each inhalation imagine you are inhaling into your being the quality of the opposite thought. For example, if your harmful thought is fear and you have identified its opposite thought as peace, imagine inhaling peace into every cell of your being with every in breath. As you exhale, imagine fear leaving your body, mind and spirit to be recycled into the Universe.

Table 6.1 Examples of replacements of harmful/ negative thoughts with opposite thoughts

Harmful/Negative thought	Potential opposite thoughts
Fear	Peace, Courage, Love
Discouraged	Strength, Assured, Confident
Hopeless	Hopeful, Expectant, Cheered
Powerless	Strong, Competent, Capable
Angry	Calm, Harmony, Love

The eight limbs

The yamas and the niyamas make up the first two limbs. The yamas are conditions of behavior, often compared to commandments, rules for living or personal guidelines. The niyamas are qualities to be cultivated, guidelines for healthy and peaceful living. Each has five parts.

The first limb—The yamas

The five yamas make up the first limb of Patanjali's eight-limbed yoga. The word yama means "restraint" or "control," but I believe that Patanjali did not mean for the yamas—or the niyamas—to be hard rules or a strict discipline. They are, like all of the sutras, meant as guides to help us become more aware and conscious. Rules simply for the sake of having rules never works to modify anyone's thinking or behavior. Becoming love, becoming compassion, union with Spirit, begins within, not through the application of stringent controls or by willpower. The yamas and niyamas are compassionate commitments to self and others. The practice begins within.

AHIMSA

The first of the yamas is ahimsa. Ahimsa is often translated to mean non-harming, non-violence, not causing pain. Sadly, human beings are often violent. Our capacity for violence of all kinds is our worst quality and greatest failing. Acknowledging our own capacity for violence—toward ourselves and others—is the beginning of change for all.

Underlying violence is almost always fear. We are regularly filled with fears, of the unknown, of others, of change. To avoid feeling our own pain, or being in pain, we often cause pain to others as a form of protection against perceived vulnerabilities. When our security is threatened on any level, our inner capacity for violence is stimulated. When any part of what we perceive as our security is at risk, we immediately begin enacting ways to stop the threat. This may take place internally or it can be an all-out fight, but it is always a form of violence. Any time we experience any amount of hostility or antagonism, inwardly or outwardly, there is violence—even if but a seed. The danger is that, when tended, seeds grow.

The experience of grief can bring with it many feelings and experiences rife with violence. Whether our loved one died violently or not, the result feels like a violation. We feel that violence has been done to us and to our beloved. We may want to lash out, to harm, to destroy. Anger or violent thoughts may fill our minds. To feel such complete powerlessness in the face of utter destruction is a pain that ultimately cannot properly be described with mere words. Often when people are filled with such despair, anger can result. We may withdraw and direct violence toward ourselves in the form of neglect, or outwardly in harmful behaviors that can damage body, mind and spirit.

Violence, inward and outward, is often a part of grief—and part of the human condition. We live in a world where anger is often more acceptable than sadness. Anger itself is not the problem, violence is the problem. Anger is a signal that there is something wrong, and when your beloved is dead, when loss has destroyed life as you knew it, there is something very wrong. Recognizing that the feelings are important and being aware of how we direct the energy of anger and fear make all the difference. Learning to replace violent and destructive feelings and tendencies with those which are loving and constructive can be difficult but it is possible.

Taking good care of yourself is essential in grief and in managing feelings of anger and fear—the seeds of violence. Yet, most of us have extreme difficulty with self-care in grief. Sometimes this is because we are so overwhelmed by the pain that we simply do not have the energy to act in a caretaking way for ourselves. Other times we may feel emotionally unable to engage in any act of love or care toward ourselves. We may feel undeserving of care or love. Because we are already in so much pain, because we may feel we do not deserve to have anything other than pain, that there can never be anything other than pain in the future in seeking to avoid the pain of grief, we often do not care about pain we may cause ourselves—no pain can be greater than the pain of being without our beloveds.

Awareness is the beginning of change. Can you observe without judgment any violence that has occurred or may be occurring inside you? Can you peel back the layers of that to see what lies beneath? Is there fear, is there anger? Where are those directed? Do you regularly perpetuate thoughts or engage in behaviors that cause harm to your body, mind, psyche or spirit? The first step to dissolving the root of violence is recognizing that it has taken root. Is there a seed that may grow? Observe with love and compassion and without judgment any violence inside you and how it manifests.

Spend some time thinking, with as much compassion as possible, about ways both large and small that you do harm to yourself. This in itself is a form of self-care. You do not have to force yourself to change your thoughts or actions, but rather attempt to become lovingly aware. Slowly and gently you can add small ways of caring for yourself. Those small ways may turn into greater acts of self-care.

Self-care is physical—taking care of your body with good food, sleep, exercise, massage, movement, sunshine and nutrition. It is mental—self-help books, music, art, creativity, seeking and finding a well-trained counselor who understands grief and bereavement. It is spiritual—in meditation, nature, study of spiritual books, chant, ritual, prayer, contemplation, speaking to a trusted religious leader. Self-care is also found in reaching out to your community—to friends and family, neighbors, co-workers; it is finding and going to a support group, to online communities. Each of these can be done with small steps forward. All of these are self-care and, with awareness and tenderness toward yourself, can grow.

SATYA

Satya is non-lying—telling the truth. It means restraining from falsehoods or distorting reality. Truth is sometimes clear, and at other times what is true may be subjective, and always, our personal truths are colored by our own perception. All of our experiences are filtered through our senses of perception, our personal system of beliefs, our opinions, ideals and values. So what is truth? And what does it mean in grief?

Truthfulness is also being genuine and congruent—living in such a way that our thoughts, feelings, words and actions are in harmony. This is yet another thing that can be difficult in grief. We live in a world that does not really understand what deep grief really means, nor what it is to live immersed in sorrow. Among other things, we are tasked with figuring out how to live authentically with and within grief, in its many forms and with its many changes and among others who may not understand. Satya's guiding principle can assist us to be mindful of living in accord with our new truth. You may feel that you are living a dual life—one in which you feel you must pretend to be okay, hiding the truth of your grief, and another private world where sadness, pain and longing may be more constant than not.

One of the biggest lies in grief is the one we tell in answer to the question, "How are you?" So often we may lie and simply say that we are fine because others are uncomfortable or, because it is socially unacceptable to cry or express sadness, we feel awkward and exposed. Occasionally, you may encounter the rare individual who wants to know, "How are you *really*?" Usually though, we believe most people don't really want to know the truth. They may be well meaning but, we think, *if they really knew the truth, they would wish they hadn't asked.*

There are many variations on "How are you?" Plunged into instant agony at the everyday questions that feel like assaults, you try to decide in a split second how or whether to answer:

"How many children do you have?"

"Are you married?"

"Can I help you?"

"Are you all right?"

"Is there something wrong?"

Do we lie or tell our truth? The pretense can be exhausting, but the lack of a safe space where the truth can simply be accepted is sorely lacking.

There are also lies of omission. Not in the classic sense of omitting specific details to intentionally deceive, but in not telling others what we want or need; by refraining from talking about our beloved, not mentioning her name, or not contributing to a conversation when the urge naturally arises. We do not do what our hearts urge us to do for many good reasons. It is painful, we may cry, others may be upset, we have received messages in the past that it is not okay to cry or to share, we don't feel safe in sharing our hearts. By not revealing ourselves, our needs, our experiences, we omit and neglect our truth. In so doing, what do we do to ourselves? Living and speaking our own personal truth is incredibly empowering. In grief, empowerment can be hard to come by.

Of course, not all situations call for total transparency and openness. With a lie or an omission, uncomfortable situations can be avoided, feelings are spared, we may seem more "together" than we really are. Sometimes that may be helpful—in a job interview or in a new situation with new people, for example. How can we know when to tell the unvarnished truth and when to keep it to ourselves?

Truth and honesty beget intimacy. The surest way to erode closeness in any relationship is dishonesty. How much truth to tell and when should be based on your level of intimacy with the person and the importance of the relationship. In your most important relationships, you must tell your truth, even if it is hard. Your most important relationship is the one you have with yourself. We must always tell the truth to ourselves. About our needs, our pain, our grief, our fears, our hopes, our dreams, our wishes.

We must tell those closest to us as much truth as we can possibly manage. When truth cannot be shared, relationships change. Intimacy erodes. When those we love and to whom we are close cannot hear our truth, even when we try to tell it, often those relationships can become sorely damaged. Sometimes relationships come to an end. Telling ourselves the truth about our relationships can be difficult.

Friends, co-workers and acquaintances should be told as much truth as is needed to maintain or to grow a connection you're comfortable with.

Strangers and those with whom you have no relationship do not necessarily need to know your deepest truths. You must judge this for yourself.

If we are to grow and become in life and in grief, we must try to be open about our truth with ourselves first and with others whom we love. This can feel risky. In grief we are extremely vulnerable. It is important to feel safe to be able to share your truth. You can begin by taking small risks. When someone asks, "How are you?", whether they mean it *really*, or whether it is social convention, you might say something like, "I'm having a hard day, but thanks for asking." This does not require the person to do or say anything further. One of the reasons many bereaved do not share how they really feel is because they do not wish to be a burden to others, to make someone else feel that they must take care of or change something. The truth is that they cannot fix this. No one can.

Another way to share your truth is be honest with yourself about what you need. If you want to talk about how you feel, if you want to hear your beloved's name, if you hope someone will reach out to you on your beloved's birthday, anniversaries, Mother's Day, Father's Day, holidays, and are afraid no one will, say so and ask for what you need. Take a risk, no matter how small, and reveal what you may feel slightly uncomfortable revealing. Practice finding comfort in the discomfort. Measure responses and determine whether it is safe to share more. If it is not safe, find a place where it is safe. Speak your truth in small doses until you feel more comfortable and empowered to do it regularly. Allow your own truth and your love to be your guide. With practice, you can hear your own inner truth, your satya, in all situations.

Asteya

Asteya means "non-stealing." *Thou shalt not steal* is the simplest way of interpreting the second yama. Most of us are not outright thieves. It is doubtful that grief drives most to steal things that don't belong to them, or to become compulsive shoplifters, though that is certainly not out of the realm of possibility. As with so much of yoga—and of life and grief—this yama can be complex. Many teachers speak of asteya as "absence of envy," "absence of jealousy" or, sometimes, "non-misappropriation"—believing that those more accurately capture the spirit of the word. The literal interpretation of non-stealing certainly can apply where appropriate. Feelings of envy, covetousness and entitlement can result in theft. We want what others have. This is a human emotion, the human condition.

Allowing envy to flourish can result in feelings of resentment, anger and injustice, even in a sense of victimhood—all of which can lead to harm to ourselves and others. Many bereaved experience the feeling of wanting what others have, which is really a form of wanting what we once had returned to us. It is a symptom of our grief. It is completely normal to feel these feelings: seemingly happy families everywhere, parents with their children, couples walking hand in hand, oblivious to the fact that in an instant it could all be gone. The pain of envy can be sharp and deep, reminding us of our own longing. Such feelings can easily turn to anger, hatred and blame—toward ourselves as well as others.

Envy is no stranger to any grieving parent who watches their dead children's friends grow, go to prom, graduate, marry, have children of their own. Weddings, graduations, births, birthday parties, family gatherings, dinners out, walking around the neighborhood, watching television—all places and occasions for tendrils of envy to unfurl from the hearts of all manner of grieving people. Mothers, fathers, widows, widowers, siblings, grandparents, friends all have experienced the feelings of envy in grief; wanting what we don't have and will never have again, desperately longing, and feeling that pain over and over.

It isn't that having these feelings is wrong in any way. They are very natural. What matters is what we do with the feelings when we notice them. Can we acknowledge them, in whatever form they come, with gentleness? Or do we swallow them, hide them even from ourselves, denying the pain and the risks inherent in such feelings. Do we feed them, and feel safer in anger, resentment and isolation than in acknowledgment of vulnerability and pain? Acknowledging envy and desire as natural results of deep grief, breathing into those spaces of hurt, allowing them to be what they are, can help them to dissipate. Let the feelings move, find a way to express them, make space for something new. To do that, we must first allow the feelings.

The foundation of envy is comparison. We divide the world into categories and classifications and compare ourselves to those on a daily basis. The more we compare, the more separate and isolated we become. Feeling isolated and separate from others increases longing for fulfillment. In grief, already feeling isolated and separate, that longing is naturally focused on our beloved dead. We envy others who are not swimming in grief, who we perceive as not tortured by such longing, we believe surely they must be more fulfilled than we. This is an understandable state of mind that in the long run does not serve us and through which we risk further separation and which can lead to harmful, violent thoughts and behavior toward ourselves and others.

Observing our thoughts and experiences mindfully, questioning our own thinking, asking ourselves if what we tell ourselves about others' fulfillment is true, witnessing our own mind with compassion and without judgment, we can continue to cultivate awareness and eventually movement toward wholeness. We can also learn to close the gap between us and others, find support and share our truths with those we can trust. Ultimately, we can return to a place where we can recognize and remember that there is no separation. Acts of comparing and envying are human constructs that serve to deepen isolation. Practicing compassion, seeking connection and always cultivating awareness can help us move more easily through painful feelings.

Brahmacharya

Brahmacharya is traditionally considered to mean celibacy, chastity or continence—holding or reining in impulses. Examining the word "continence" and its meaning can offer a broader way to apply the concept of this yama. Perhaps, like so much in the *Sutras*, it means more than one thing.

Swami Satchidananda's commentary on brahmacharya discusses the practice as the conservation of life energy, of not becoming depleted. He further discusses brahmacharya as resulting in the preservation of *virya*, which translates to mean "vital energy." Mukunda Stiles in his interpretation of the *Sutras* translates brahmacharya to mean "behavior that respects the Divine as omnipresent." As a tantrik, Mukunda believed and taught that the Divine is present in all. Behaving in ways which honor the Divine presence everywhere at all times with reverence, including within our own physical form, would naturally result in treating our bodies, and those of others, respectfully, as temples of Spirit and manifestations of the Divine.

As in all of yoga, being aware of our behavior and how it impacts us, those we love and the world around us is fundamental. Brahmacharya, seen as restraint of impulses—continence—may be a more useful and expansive way of understanding and practicing this yama. Practicing even a moment of restraint before engaging in impulsive, harmful or avoidant behavior allows some space in which to examine ourselves and our motives. We may also use that moment for practice of the other yamas, satya and ahimsa—truthfulness and non-violence. We can observe whether we are being honest with ourselves about our behavior and its root causes, and whether it is harmful.

Why do so many of us engage in harmful, avoidant or impulsive behavior in grief? Traumatic grief is trauma. This seems obvious, but for so many it is not. Trauma involves a deeply distressing or disturbing occurrence that impacts our entire being. The effects of trauma can be long term and are stored in our physical, mental and energy bodies—all of the first three koshas—annamaya kosha, pranamaya kosha and manomaya kosha.

Trauma and grief are incredibly stressful events. When you live with grief and trauma, your physical body is almost always in a state of stress, the levels of which can vary moment to moment. The body's stress response is a normal reaction to a threatening situation. It is part of our nervous system and works automatically when the brain perceives potential harm—the classic "fight or flight" response.

In most cases, when we are stressed, we do not engage in combat or run away because either of those is usually inappropriate. We instead freeze. We become still and stiff, rather than use muscles primed for action. We often suppress emotional reactions. Because the stress is never truly discharged, it lies just beneath the surface. Our bodies and minds are primed to quickly recall the unsafe or stressful states that created the trauma and any similar events easily and quickly triggering the stress response again. And the cycle repeats itself.

Over time, we begin seeking ways to numb and distract ourselves from a near perpetual state of stress. Seeking relief from chronic tension, we often take medication, drink alcohol or use other substances. We engage in all manner of distraction to attempt to cope with pain and discomfort. Reflect for a moment on the various ways you distract yourself from vulnerability, pain, emotional upheaval and near constant stress.

Make a list in your journal, or even just in your mind. What do you use to avoid experiencing pain and stress? Do you shop, eat, drink, take drugs (prescribed or otherwise), work, run, have sex, argue, exercise, pray, go to church, watch TV, gossip, cook, start drama, stay busy, take on another project, paint, knit, read? Whatever your ways of coping and distracting—do you use these things appropriately and mindfully? What things on your list are causing harm to you? Even seemingly non-harmful things when overused or used mindlessly can cause harm. When we consistently unconsciously avoid in order to evade reality and its inherent pain, we eventually find ourselves in further pain.

In practicing brahmacharya, we can begin to cultivate the ability to pay closer attention to our impulses. We can be honest with ourselves about whether indulging may be depleting our vital energy, strength, focus or will. When you have an impulse to do whatever it is you do to avoid discomfort, simply notice. See if you can restrain the impulse if only for a moment and simply be with the discomfort.

Explore what is beneath by asking questions of yourself, "Why am I pouring this drink?" or "What am I avoiding by mindlessly watching TV?" or "Do I really want to share my body with this person and why?" or "What am I seeking to numb by taking this pill?" Stop and notice, then try to focus your attention on your breath and your body. Allow yourself a space to be with the feeling, if only for a few seconds. Notice whether you feel different; is the impulse stronger or has it waned? No judgment, simply noticing. What can you do in a mindful way that will conserve and increase your vital energy, your virya? Can you practice restraint lovingly, even for a moment? This practice can shift the balance toward sattva, harmony. That is brahmacharya.

Aparigraha

Aparigraha is usually translated as the absence of greed. It also translates to mean non-grasping or non-attachment. The two have similar root causes, but they are not exactly the same. We can be intensely aware of our attachments and at the same time not grasp. Generally when there is grasping, there is attachment, but where there is attachment there is not always grasping.

Non-attachment in grief is one of the most difficult and painful concepts to wrap our minds around. A grieving person certainly would not be grieving if he didn't have an attachment to his beloved who has died, or attachment to the relationship that has been lost. But attachments are not easy to release. Just as everything else in the yamas, we can't simply cease our feelings or our behavior, at least for very long, by sheer willpower. It involves practice.

The Buddha taught that attachment is the cause of suffering. It is one thing to know that and another to simply release attachment. The Buddha also taught that the reasons for suffering are craving and ignorance. A grieving heart craves the presence, the touch, the smell, the sound, the sight of the beloved who is missing. That kind of attachment is difficult to transcend. Grasping comes when we attempt to appease the craving with something else—possessions, control, money, status, other people. And when we do this in ignorance, with no understanding of why or what we are doing, it can be harder and harder to relax the grasp.

You may wish to revisit the Bhakti chapter and read the section on padma and samputa mudras (Figures 3.7 and 3.8 on pages 97 and 98), the description and practices of which address attachment and identification as well as separating ego grasping from love. The love, the reason for our attachment to our beloveds, need never be released. Practicing the heart mudras in that section can help us to release and relax any form of attachments or grasping which no longer serve, while nurturing the love we hold for our beloveds and cultivating it also for ourselves.

Practice of aparigraha can help us examine ways that grasping can arise from attachment. The notion of grasping carries with it a sense of reaching, of holding on desperately, also of seeking to control. The perceived need for control plays a role in grief. How many of us have witnessed greed and control rear their ugly heads after the death of a loved one? Grasping, greed and possessiveness are often painful sources of conflict for families, sometimes even before death arrives. End of life issues, whether to call the hospice, whether to cease life-prolonging measures, whether to cremate or bury, and who gets what, are all too familiar to many families.

Greed and grasping come from a place of fear, of pain and of "not enough." Some family members may feel that an inheritance is "rightly" theirs and have deep attachment to an identity—favored child, firstborn, next in line to the throne. Others may grasp for physical items—jewelry, heirlooms, houses—because these belonged to their loved one, because they are the source of treasured memories and to release the object may feel like releasing memories, or even the beloved deceased. Some want power or as much money as possible. That kind of greed also comes from a place of fear and the mistaken belief that money, possessions and power over others somehow ensures security, safety and the preservation or continuity of self.

With the experience of deep grief often comes a fear of losing other loved ones. Anxiety and grief are intimately linked. When we realize what we can lose, knowing how incredibly painful and helpless it feels, fearing the deaths of others we love and cherish is completely normal. But normal or not, this feeling can be paralyzing. When we feel this kind of fear, we may seek all manner of ways to alleviate it. We may attempt to control our environments or even other people in the attempt to feel secure.

Yoga teaches us that this kind of thinking is ego-based—meaning that it is the ego, the "I-maker," *ahamkara*, seeking continuity. It is our ego, our sense of "I" and "me" that seeks to grasp onto things and people and situations, out of fear that if these things change, we no longer have the ones we love, to care for, to nurture, to grow with and live with. The reality is that many people who have experienced traumatic grief and loss know we control almost nothing, though we certainly try. Sometimes the trying creates more pain for us than the grief itself.

It's not hard to recognize that the opposite of grasping is releasing. Just let go, let her go, let him go, let the feelings go, let the fear and the anger go, say goodbye, move on. It is nearly impossible to just simply "let it go," though the bereaved often hear it in some form or other—from family, friends, doctors, therapists, religious leaders. This is not helpful. The practice of aparigraha—non-grasping—begins first with simply recognizing that we may be grasping. And then, what, where and why we may be grasping—and then perhaps, little by little, we can release some of the tension. We begin by simply noticing.

It isn't that we *shouldn't* be attached. We *are* attached. We have attachment. Seeing it openly, without judgment, simply as it is—that is the practice. We are attached because ego seeks continuity in our loved ones and in ourselves. Our attachment is in everything our beloveds were and are and what they continue to represent to us. Author Stephen K. Levine says, "Suffering is wanting to be something other than what we are or wanting to be someplace other than where we are" (p.142). To tell a deeply grieving person that they need to just let that go makes no sense whatsoever.

But what we can do is see it. Be aware of it and as much as possible, be open to feeling it. And I'm not even saying you should *want* to do that. That profound definition of suffering also counts when we want to not be suffering and suffering is what is happening. When we want the pain gone and it's not. When we *want* to let go and cannot. When we want them to never have died and they did. Wanting something to be different is to suffer. Allowing whatever is to simply be is to move a little closer to freedom from grasping when we suffer. Whether that is an intense fear of death, a fear of losing everything and everyone, a fear of being penniless, a fear of having nothing, a fear of being alone, of being wrong, of being anything at all other that what we are in this very moment keeps us simply from *being*. Becoming aware, noticing and surrendering as much as you can, to what is—this is the practice of aparigraha.

The second limb—The niyamas

The niyamas are the next limb in Patanjali's Ashtanga yoga. They complement the Yamas and are generally referred to as "observances." Where the yamas are filled with things that we are to refrain from doing, the Niyamas are things we are to do, to practice and to cultivate in our lives. They are guides for how to treat yourself in body, mind, energy and spirit.

Saucha

Saucha is most often translated as cleanliness. It is also interpreted as purity. I believe its definition envelops all aspects of self-care. Cleanliness isn't just about removing the physical dirt, clutter and mess from our homes or workspaces, it is also about removing dirt, clutter and mess from our minds, our bodies and our energy fields. To work toward giving ourselves clean spaces, healthy bodies, clear minds and pure fields of energy, is to treat ourselves with kindness and compassion, believing ourselves worthy of care.

Particularly in times of traumatic and early grief, we may find it difficult to care for ourselves. Acts such as taking showers, dressing, doing laundry, going to work, seem useless activities that mean absolutely nothing. Why should you bother? Why do these things matter? To not care about these things is normal in the abnormal circumstance of suddenly having to live with the knowledge that your beloved is dead and will be so for the rest of all of your tomorrows.

When one is in the depths of grief, it is okay to have trouble doing these things. Those things do not make sense. Eventually doing such things will make sense again. If you are having a lot of trouble, ask for help from someone you trust. If someone offers help, accept their help, even if you don't know what you need. If someone suggests taking a shower or a long hot bath, do it. It will help you to relax and to feel more human, even if you don't care to feel human right now. Why should anyone in a traumatically bereaved state care that they may smell bad, or that they once wore makeup, or ate food or cleaned things? Eventually you will begin to take steps toward doing these things again. For now you may not feel that you have enough time, love, space, support, help or permission to feel and express what you are feeling so that you can find your way through the pain. If you can find a way to have more of those things, you will more easily find your way.

Saucha can be practiced inwardly as well as outwardly, in giving the body nourishment with good food and working to purify the body of toxins. In grief, changes in appetite are very common, some people turn to high sugar, high fat foods for comfort, or as a stress response. Others may neglect nutrition by not eating at all. We may ingest other toxins that are not good for body and mind, such as alcohol and drugs (prescribed or not) that may cloud thinking or reduce the ability to truly experience what we are feeling. You might consider the practice of brahmacharya, restraint of impulses, when you feel the need to have another soda or another vodka. You might add just one meal a day of good healthy veggies. You might think of meeting with an herbalist or a naturopath for help in choices for cleansing and detoxifying herbs and foods to best support your koshas.

If you can, schedule a massage on a regular basis to help release toxins and tension from the body. Drink water to stay hydrated and flush toxins from the body. Practice asana daily. A few sun salutations or even just one or two poses a day can help your body release tension and toxins, give more freedom of movement and shift your mental space. Pay attention to sleep. Restful sleep in trauma and grief can be hard to come by. How is your sleep? How can you get better rest? Speak to a reputable aromatherapist about essential oils that have a relaxing and sedative effect, drink chamomile or valerian root tea before bed. Speak to your healthcare practitioner about whether melatonin might work for you. Acupuncture treatments may help insomnia, and never underestimate the power of a warm bath.

Clearing our chakras in pranamaya kosha can be helpful as well. This is also self-care. Take ritual baths with sea salts and essential oils that can help clear your energy, refresh your spirit and bring some calm and perhaps a sense of peace. Research ways to balance chakra function. You may wish to see an energy healer, reiki practitioner, acupuncturist or other practitioner of Traditional Chinese Medicine. Get sunlight daily. The sun purifies the mind as well as the energy field and is a direct source of prana. Visit bodies of water if this is possible.

Practice purity of mind through meditation, reading inspirational books, listening to music that you find uplifting and which help you honor where you are in your grief. Surround yourself with images of things that you find uplifting and beautiful—art, family photos, statues of your chosen deities, and any other art that lifts your spirit and calms your mind. Bring plants and flowers into your environment. Plants help purify the air as well as lend some of their own prana to the space that they are dwelling in. Take a media break and stay away from news or social media for a while. Saucha moves us toward a state of balance and harmony, which is the yogic goal of sattva, balance.

Santosha

Santosha means contentment. This is often a difficult niyama for a grieving person to cultivate. It may not even seem possible in early or traumatic grief, at least for a long while. What is contentment? Most people agree that contentment includes a sense of peace, of quiet satisfaction, mostly independent of external circumstances. Contentment isn't the same thing as happiness, which a transient emotion. Contentment and inner peace can be far more lasting.

In grief, finding a place of contentment can be extremely difficult. Our inner space is full of pain. We are questioning, raging, weeping, confused, yearning and longing for what we cannot have. A great part of yoga in grief is in cultivating our ability to accommodate these feelings, adapt to these feelings, adjust our inner and outer lives to the grief state. When we are discontent, yoga asks us to notice, to be gentle with ourselves, to see if we can sit with the feelings and notice again if they shift. It is okay if they don't, it is okay if they do. Yoga asks us also, when we are ready, to begin to cultivate those things which help us to adapt, adjust and accommodate further.

Cultivating contentment can help with this. Cultivation of anything requires first observation and care in taking steps for preparation. When we want to grow a garden, we first look for the best place to begin. Then we cultivate the soil so that what we plant will grow. Cultivating contentment, or any other quality in the niyamas, is the same. We first observe and then take small steps to begin to care for ourselves so we can grow new things. Growth doesn't happen overnight.

In a support group of bereaved parents, one grieving mother, 11 years into the deep grief that followed the accidental death of her teen daughter, talked about her practice of cultivating contentment, how she accepts moments of santosha when they come, "wrapping them around me, like a cloak of contentment." She spoke of working on allowing that contentment to stay as long as possible when it came. Parents only months past the traumatic deaths of their children could not even fathom what she was talking about. And nor should they. We are all on our own journeys. Another mother later in the group shared the immense anger and hatred she was feeling—even toward inanimate objects simply because they existed, and her two children did not. Contentment was nowhere in sight.

There's something to be learned though from the notion of holding on to even fleeting moments of contentment when they arise. Think about what contentment means to you. How might it show up? Can you allow a moment of peace, satisfaction or calm to be as it is for however long it may last? Allowing moments of contentment when they come can be a challenge for many in grief. One sister whose identical twin died of a rare cancer shared how difficult it is for her to hold on to moments of peace when they come. When she notices a sense of contentment, the profound sadness at all that her twin will never, see, do or feel again overtakes the peace almost immediately. Even though she has become very practiced at feeling whatever she is feeling, she expresses how much more difficult it is to hold and experience the good feelings when they come.

Contentment is good. We know that feeling content, peaceful, relaxed and satisfied is good. None of these are things we can simply will into being. But we can learn to cultivate them, and if not to hold them, to perhaps appreciate them when they come, no matter how fleeting they may be. One of the most significant ways of doing this is by experiencing the present moment as it is as often as possible. Where ever you are, whatever you are doing, is it possible to stop and fully experience your surroundings? Try it now. Take a breath and notice the wonder of your own breath, how your body moves as the oxygen comes in and goes out. Close your eyes and notice your heartbeat, any sense of energy in your body, any heaviness or lightness that is there. Opening your eyes, look at your surroundings noticing fully what is there, noticing how this very moment contains so much that we normally do not recognize or see. Notice the book you may be holding in your hands, how many people all over the world participated in its making, how it came to you where you are at this very moment. Can a practice of mindfulness of your experience in this present moment lead to something like contentment in this present moment? And if it can, even for the briefest period, can we allow it to be what it is?

The practice of noticing without judgment a sense of content or discontent, and allowing it to be or to fade can help us to cultivate our ability to be in the moment with what is. Even if contentment may not be available, when fleeting moments of satisfaction, appreciation or gratitude appear, is it possible to notice and fully experience those without judgment as well? And can they bring you a bit closer to contentment? Even for that brief moment? Simply notice.

TAPAS

The root *tap* is central to any form of Sanskrit word having to do with warmth or heat. Throughout the Vedic scriptures not only does the word have to do with the more widespread notions of tapas as austerity and asceticism, but also with the most basic of all human needs, simple warmth. The idea of warmth conjures images of a cozy fire, comfort food, the warm hand of a friend, of safety and security. In order to become more comfortable in our discomfort, we must first feel safe. The idea of accepting tapas as pain in order to move toward transformation is positively untenable if you do not have a sense of safety.

The Vedic scriptures speak of the tapas of the sun, the tapas and the heat of life and the warmth necessary to new growth—the hatching of new life is compared to the heat of the Cosmic life force that animates all existence. Tapas is the heat, the light, the warmth that allows all life to thrive and to grow. It is the constant burning of the sun, it is energy, it is fuel, it is that which spurs us on and beckons us to turn our face toward rather than away. It is heat generated in the body from movement, the heat that is made when the body converts food to energy, the heat and energy that builds to create and grow anything at all: a vegetable garden, babies, love, flowers, friendship, a new business. What warmth, what heat do you need in your life right now to help you grow and thrive from this place where you are now?

Tapas also means to burn, to purify. It is in a sense its own kind of alchemy. Before Patanjali discusses the niyamas, he speaks of tapas in the first sutra of Book II, The Portion on Practice, sutra 2:1: *Tapah svadhyaya esvara pranidhanani kriya yoga*. Swami Satchidananda in his translation and commentary of the sutras (2003) interprets this to mean, "Accepting pain as help for purification, study of spiritual books, and surrender to the Supreme Being constitute Yoga in practice" (p.79). In this opening sutra, Patanjali tells us that these three niyamas—tapas, svadhyaya and ishvara pranidhana—essentially are yoga in practice.

The notion of receiving pain, tapas, from the Universe, from God, in whatever form it may take as an instrument of purification and spiritual transformation is a challenging one. It makes a good bit of sense though. Here we are in it. Running from it doesn't help. Avoiding it doesn't make it go away. In fact, when we avoid, we serve only to exponentially increase the pain, to create new pain, or at the very least, we find ourselves ill prepared to manage the pain when it takes us by surprise. When we practice turning willingly toward the pain, when we engage with the pain when it comes, eventually we find that it no longer has the capacity to run us completely off into the ditch. Attempts to avoid painful thoughts, feelings, memories, sensations, serve only to ease the pain temporarily and ultimately keep us from living fully and growing forward in our lives.

When we can willingly move into our own pain and grief, including uninvited stress brought on by triggers—in the grocery store, on TV, at social events, at the doctor's office, in line at the post office—wherever we are, whatever we're doing, these things become less and less able to derail us. And from the pain comes growth and meaning, which is what all of humanity is seeking. This is the benefit, and even the gift, of tapas in grief, loss and trauma.

In order to be able to approach our pain, to engage, to not turn away, to accept tapas when it comes, as it comes, we must first begin with compassion and gentleness toward ourselves. The entire practice of yoga, everything that has been discussed here and in previous chapters, states over and over in different ways the necessity of mindfulness and awareness without judgment and with compassion in order to integrate our pain and the experience of the loss. We must have compassion toward ourselves to be able to withstand pain in a healthy and meaningful way. We must cultivate self-compassion and self-love. Where love and compassion exist, fear and pain are dissolved.

Turning away from pain ensures that we continue to live only in bits and pieces, in fear, fragmented, disjointed and distressed. By remembering, honoring and being with the pain we integrate the experience into the whole of who we are. In order to first tolerate and then willingly incorporate the pain, we must have an experience of safety. How can you increase your sense of safety even in your pain? As you increase your ability to tolerate the sensations that come when the pain and the memories come, you increase your own store of tapas which lends you strength. Like the heat built when we lift a physical weight over and over again, the spiritual and emotional weight of grief and pain when lifted, carried and experienced safely, consciously causes those metaphoric muscles to become stronger and more able to endure the heat of burning. This is the secret to living with grief. You never figure out how to make it go away and you don't get over it; you eventually become conditioned to better carry the weight. And in the carrying, the weight itself can even be transformed.

The side-effect and the benefit of this kind of tapas is that in so many ways, as we become stronger in our own experiences, we become better able to help others carry the weight when they are not yet strong. Viktor Frankl (2006), the great Austrian psychiatrist and Holocaust survivor said, "What is to give light, must endure burning" (p.69). That burning is tapas.

Svadhyaya

Classically, svadhyaya is the study of sacred and spiritual texts. It also translates to mean study of self and self-reflection. It is gaining knowledge of ourselves through not only spiritual texts, spiritual leaders and masters, but also through observing our own behaviors, reactions, habitual ways of being, questioning why we do what we do, or don't do what we don't do.

The practice and cultivation of svadhyaya helps us to learn to find our own answers. When we read a sacred text, or listen to an inspirational sermon or dharma talk, when we sit at the feet of a master teacher or guru, we can learn, but only in applying that knowledge to the self can we find our own truth. This is the crucial difference between information and knowledge. Svadhyaya is very closely related to the self-inquiry processes of Jnana yoga, underscoring once more how all the practices are related. When we spend time in self-reflection, noticing things about ourselves and our lives in compassionate ways, we can become more empowered to change the things that we can see need to be changed in order for continued growth. As a dear teacher once told me, when we are in a process of self-inquiry and engaged in the practice of svadhyaya, doors are always opening. This is the opposite of the experiences we have when we are in a place of avoidance and ignorance. When we evade the truth of ourselves, our behavior, our motivations, our habits and the impact of those on ourselves and those around us, our world is made smaller.

Because grief and loss are spiritual crises, cultivation of svadhyaya in these circumstances can be difficult and painful. A natural unfolding of a spiritual crisis includes the questioning of values and beliefs, of examining and re-examining the constructs that we once believed to be solid. C.S. Lewis in *A Grief Observed* (1996) writes:

> You never know how much you really believe anything until its truth or falsehood becomes a matter of life and death to you. It is easy to say you believe a rope to be strong and sound as long as you are merely using it to cord a box. But suppose you had to hang by that rope over a precipice. Wouldn't you then first discover how much you really trusted it? (p.22)

A spiritual crisis brings many to that place of the precipice. We question God, the meaning of life, the loss and all secondary losses, the why and the how; we question who we are, and who we are not, now that this has happened. Everything we thought we knew seems completely useless, devoid of meaning. We must find and make meaning elsewhere. When everything outside of us is no longer what it once was, and everything we thought solid is no longer, the only other place to look is on the inside. Looking inward can be difficult. We may read sacred texts we once found comforting only to find that truth we once saw there is now distorted. Or that it makes us angry, that it says something completely different from what we thought it said before. This may spur us to read, see and think in different ways; we may form new or altered personal meanings. We may seek new spiritual guidance elsewhere—or nowhere. We may have no idea where to begin to look. A spiritual crisis has nothing to do with religion or dogma. It is an internal and wholly individual experience which stimulates a desire to find and make meaning of loss, of pain, and of the rest of our lives as they must be lived in this way. The practice of svadhyaya helps us navigate spiritual crisis and find direction.

Finding teachers, guides and appropriate material for reading and listening is an individual process that must be based on your own personal and spiritual needs. I include all manner of material in my definition of spiritual and sacred texts. You may resonate with traditional sacred texts of various religious and spiritual paths, like the Holy Bible, the Rig Veda, the Upanishads, the Bhagavad Gita, the Talmud, the Koran, the Mahayana Sutras, the Tao Te Ching, but there are many other sacred and spiritual writings: The Tibetan Book of the Dead, the Gnostic gospels, the works of Rumi, Khalil Gabran, St. Teresa of Avila, St. Francis, St. John of the Cross and, of course, Patanjali. Pagan beliefs are discussed in *The Golden Bough*, *The White Goddess* and the collected works of Margaret Murray. To me, Shakespeare's writing is sacred, and certainly teaches spiritual truths. There are a plethora of spiritual lessons in the world of fiction of all kinds. The works of more modern day teachers and writers can deliver a great deal of spiritual wisdom even when the material is secular. There is much to be found in theater, poetry, prose, art and music. Meditation, prayer, chant, movement and connecting with nature all help us to practice svadhyaya.

If we do not feel inspired at all by sacred and spiritual texts, where else can we cultivate inspiration? If we can no longer find God, Goddess, Spirit where we used to be able to find It/Her/Him, where else might you find that Divine Spirit? If you feel you cannot connect directly to God through spiritual texts or spiritual teachers, spend some time in svadhyaya's other aspect— self-reflection. Find a safe, warm, comfortable, calming space and move your awareness inward. Take a few deep centering and calming breaths. Imagine breathing into your heart space, opening that field, and ask yourself this: "When I cannot connect directly to God, what are the things around me that inspire me? In what other things can I see God?"

Is it nature, animals, other people? Is it in a feeling like hope, peace or courage? Is it laughter, music or art? What else brings you a sense of inspiration? Is there one thing you can do to deepen your own personal connection with that connecting thing? This is also svadhyaya. Instead of focusing on what God is not, think of what God *is* to you—and grow experiences of those qualities and experiences in your life. This helps to grow your spirit and deepen self-awareness, which is the function of svadhyaya.

ISHVARA PRANIDHANA

We end the niyamas with ishvara pranidhana—surrender. From tapas to svadhyaya to ishvara pranidhana, the progression is a continuum. The pain and spiritual crisis of grief is ultimately about surrender. As mentioned earlier with the discussion of the opening sutra: "Tapas, svadhyaya, ishvara pranidhana constitute yoga in practice." The three are interrelated. Through tapas, we are able to see and face the pain and truth of our lives. Through svadhyaya, we come to realize that we cannot continually endure the pain that comes with life and death on our own. Which leads then to, as Mukunda Stiles puts it, "a process of gradually unveiling the form of the Divine that is of your choosing and that is attracted to you. In this manner, a personal relationship with the subtlest of forms begins" (p.115). This is ishvara pranidhana. Divine "omnipresence, omnipotence, and omniscience begin to comfort and guide you in all areas." We move into that space through surrender.

Surrender is not about giving up. It is a way of moving toward, of leaning in. Leaning, as much as we possibly can, into the pain, the challenges, the doubt, the anxiety, the fear, the hurt, the changing tides of emotions and of uncertainty. Also leaning into pleasure, laughter, enjoyment and happiness—even if you feel you shouldn't or that you do not deserve it. Accepting the grace of santosha, contentment, when it comes, you can find the inner strength to continue to lean in and forward, extending your comfort zone, testing your edges, moving more deeply into a space of love and interconnectedness. That movement, the journey through and inward, takes us all closer and closer to Yoga, to pure Union, toward *samadhi*, Divine consciousness.

The idea of surrender can bring with it opposing feelings of relief and opposition in equal measure. To surrender is to release control. This is uncomfortable because we believe that if we remain in control, we can stave off pain, relieve anxiety, and ultimately stop bad things from happening. But this is not true. We can never really stop bad things from happening. We can do our very best to take care of ourselves and others, but ultimately we must release the notion that we control anything other than ourselves and our own reactions, responses and behaviors.

In a recent conversation with a deeply grieving woman, she spoke of desperately wanting a break from her grief. And she deserved a break after multiple miscarriages, the death of her infant son, the death of her grandmother, an aunt, her cat and, only days earlier, her beloved dog. She wept and wondered aloud who would be next. We discussed the fear that comes with that, and the not knowing, and how we manage it—how do we manage the sense of unfairness, the pain, the uncertainty, the fear, the weariness of grief? Only in surrender can we truly find peace.

Surrender means to cease a struggle or fight, it also means to give over; it is an act of submission and of yielding. Ishvara means "Supreme Being" and carries the special connotation of meaning not only The One Supreme Being, but also one's own personal deity. Ishvara is your very own personal, private, individually unique notion of the Divine with whom you have your own unique relationship. To what supreme force would you, could you, do you surrender your all? Recall our discussion in the svadhyaya section about cultivation of what God *is* for you in your life. In what ways do you find and see what God *is* within your life and in the world, rather than what God is not? How would you cultivate those qualities of Divinity? In the cultivation of those is also the key to surrender. Svadhyaya leads to surrender.

The ultimate force of Divinity is love. When we see that God is truly Love, that we are all truly Love, we can far more easily release our constant battle *against*—against circumstances, against grief, against pain, against God, against anything—and surrender. We can be soft and yielding. In that state, we can absorb and expand infinitely. This is the opposite of being hard, the antithesis of resisting, deflecting, defending or controlling. We can open, accept and receive. This causes us to be full, rather than depleted. And the more we are filled, the more fully we can become and be who we truly are.

Ultimately, surrender is about releasing any and all energies and thoughts that are not based in love. Love surrenders all. Love always surrenders. Spiritual teacher Marianne Williamson in her book, *Return to Love* (1996) says this about surrender:

> Something amazing happens when we surrender and just love. We melt into another world, a realm of power already within us. The world changes when we change. The world softens when we soften. The world loves us when we choose to love the world. (p.61)

Our grief softens, our hearts soften, our responses soften, our prickly places soften. We become like Love.

Meditation

Surrender to the heart of love

Come into a comfortable seated position, either cross-legged on the floor, on a cushion or seated in a supportive chair. Find a way of sitting that is completely supported and comfortable.

Let the spine be long and tall, but not stiff. You may wish to roll the shoulders up toward the ears, back and down, creating a more open chest and heart space. Let your hands be relaxed or, if you wish, cross the palms over the heart center, or take anjali mudra. Take a few deep breaths into the belly to center and relax and allow your breathing to return to normal.

Imagine that as you breathe in, you are literally breathing in and out through your heart. Imagine your heart and the energetic field around your heart growing fuller and softer with each breath. If you wish, you can repeat with each inhalation, either mentally or softly aloud, "I surrender..." and on each out breath, "...to Love." Continue with each breath to imagine the breath and the prana moving in and out of your heart space, not through the power of your lungs, but by the power of your heart. Imagine that the field of love continues to grow larger and larger, extending infinitely throughout the universe. You may notice a building of warmth, a sense of fullness, an expansion or a sense of release. Feel the energy of Love surrounding and permeating your koshas and the space around you. Allow Love to absorb and dissolve any feelings of pain, of anger, of confusion, of tension, of stress, of worry—anything that you may be carrying that is not of love and which you would like to release. This is surrender.

The third limb—Asana

Asana is the third limb of Patanjali's Raja yoga. Patanjali clearly states in sutra 2:46, "*Sthira sukham asanam.*" This says: "Asana is a steady, comfortable posture" (Swami Satchidanauda). The posture should always be comfortable and bring with it a sense of steadiness. In the following sutra, 2:47, he tells us that asana is "mastered by relaxation of effort, to create a lessening of the natural tendency for restlessness" (Mukunda Stiles). In grief, often even in states of extreme weariness and exhaustion, we carry a sense of restlessness. When our beloved has died, when we have been through trauma, when our lives are rocked by the devastation of loss, a deep sense of restlessness often fills our hearts, minds and bodies. Finding a place of rest in grief can seem impossible at times. The practice of asana works against that restless tendency to help bring a sense of steadiness and comfort. In a sense it's another form of surrender.

Asana and many specific yoga postures will be covered in depth in the chapter on Hatha yoga. Asana works on the physical body, annamaya kosha, as well as on the energy body, pranamaya kosha, to help calm and still the restlessness of the mind, manomaya kosha. There are myriad physical benefits of asana practice, but it is the energetic, mental and spiritual aspect of asana practice that makes it different from any other physical exercise. The various yoga postures create changes and benefits to cardiovascular function and musculoskeletal structure, including strengthening muscles and increasing flexibility and balance. It increases circulation and helps decrease toxins in the body, particularly together with breathwork. All of these can help with the physical challenges of grief as well as many of the mental and emotional aspects.

Yoga masters say that even the mastery of one yoga posture will bring the benefit of yoga—the relaxation of effort and steadiness of body leading to stillness and the sense of transcendence beyond dualities. This eventual state creates a sense of wholeness and unity with all, which is the overall goal of yoga.

The fourth limb—Pranayama

Prana means "life force" and yama means "control," so the word literally means "control of life force." Because one of the main ways that we bring prana into our bodies is through the breath, pranayama appears to be breathwork. Ultimately the practices are about moving and controlling the prana throughout our koshas by way of the breath, as well as during meditation practices.

Prana was also discussed in the Koshas section of the Tantra chapter. The second layer of our being is pranamaya kosha, the sheath made of prana— our life force energy. If you haven't yet read that chapter or section, please do in order to have a better understanding of prana and what we are doing when we practice pranayama. Within pranamaya kosha are our energetic centers, the chakras. Prana and the pranamaya kosha is the bridge between the physical body and the mind. This is why when we are anxious or upset we can use the breath to calm the body and help focus the mind. Pranayama practices help to detoxify the physical body and to balance, recharge and illuminate the energetic, subtle bodies.

When pranayama is mastered, the sense of the movement of prana is evident and one can sense the prana permeating the koshas. Patanjali tells us in sutra 2:49 that pranayama extends naturally from asana. In sutra 2:50 Patanjali tells us that we can practice pranayama by inhalation, exhalation, and by retention of the breath. He says pranayama is to be regulated by location of the breath in the body, the amount of time which we breathe in, out, or retain the breath, or by how many breaths we take in any specific practice, "regulated by space, time, or number, long or short." He tells us in sutra 2:51 that there is a fourth kind of pranayama which occurs during concentration on an internal or external object. When the mind comes to a place of complete stillness, so does the prana. It ceases movement and fully saturates our being, being preserved in our koshas and tissues.

Grief requires a lot of energy and depletes our koshas on the levels of annamaya (physical), pranamaya (energetic), and manomaya (mind) koshas. Practicing Raja yoga and particularly pranayama can help replace much of the energy that is expended in the process of grief. Specific practices for pranayama are discussed in the Hatha yoga chapter.

The fifth limb—Pratyahara

Pratyahara is most often translated to mean "withdrawal of the senses." The Sanskrit *ahara* means "anything taken from outside ourselves." *Prati* is a preposition that means "against" or "to remove." Pratyahara, then, is the removal of external objects, influences and stimuli. More rarely discussed than almost any of the other eight limbs, pratyahara is essential in movement to the next limb in the practices of Raja. Some teachers include pratyahara as part of Hatha yoga practices—those which have to do with the physical body—and some include it as an inner practice. It is actually both of these. Pratyahara is the bridge that teaches us to move from the outer world to the inner world and more readily into a space of concentration and meditation.

Many people who say they "can't meditate" say this because they think that they cannot quiet the mind. The mind races and runs due to sensory input of all kinds. In yogic teachings, there are three kinds of ahara. The first is literally food that we feed our physical bodies. The second is information we receive, register and interpret through our physical senses—the classic five: sound, sight, taste, touch, smell, as well as the other four lesser-known senses that detect heat and cold (thermoception), pain (nociception), balance and movement (equilbrioception/vestibular) and the sense of body awareness (proprioception). The third kind of ahara includes the sensory impressions we experience in relationship to others and how we take in and react to the energies that result from those connections.

In our twenty-first-century world we may believe it more difficult than ever to find space and time to quiet the senses and move inward. Surely we have far more sensory distractions than did the ancients; they didn't have to deal with email, smart phones, traffic jams, CNN, Fox News, malls, social media, on-demand culture, nearly unlimited quantities of sugar, salt, fat, preservatives, additives, a plethora of consciousness altering substances and all manner of things that are not very good for the body, mind or spirit available at the touch of a button, the stroke of a key or the slide of a debit card. But as these teachings exist and are spoken of throughout spiritual texts of myriad paths, this must have been a human problem for some time.

The dangers of the inability to release attachment to the senses is described in the *Upanishads* using the metaphor of a chariot (our physical body) that carries a precious passenger (our True Self). The chariot is pulled by powerful horses (our senses) and driven by an intelligent driver (*bhuddi*/wisdom) who must learn to use the reins (the mind/manas) wisely and carefully in order to control the horses properly. If the horses are not trained properly, or they lose control, if the driver is untrained or distracted, the chariot will end up off course, somewhere other than it was meant to be or, at worst, crashed on the side of the road. The True Self will of course be fine, but that's probably not how we want the journey to go.

In grief, it is not unusual to experience sensory changes in the way we perceive the world around us. It can be very helpful to know that sometimes difficult or traumatic experiences can create stress that might cause changes or differences in sensory perception and processing. You may notice changes in how you see or hear things—colors or patterns may seem brighter and bigger, sounds may seem louder, more difficult to separate. You may notice differences in ways that your body responds to touch or sensations of pressure. You may become easily overwhelmed in busy or loud places, be unable to tolerate a lot of sensory information at once or simply have no patience for meaningless chit-chat. The ringing of a telephone may send you into a meltdown; the sound of voices or a dog barking may trigger a headache or extreme agitation. You may find that you suddenly have difficulty maintaining eye contact. This may all sound strange, but these are not uncommon experiences for trauma survivors or those in traumatic and deep grief. These experiences can increase fear and anxiety in grief and can greatly impact your ability to function in your day-to-day life.

As discussed previously, anxiety is a large part of grief. Anxiety, as well as other painful emotional responses, is often triggered by our sensory perceptions—something we see, hear, smell, remember, think. In grief, we are almost always under stress. Learning to calm and withdraw the responses of the senses can help to ease stress and help bridge the way to meditation, which can allow the fluctuations of the mind to cease and lead to Union.

In a heightened state of stress, the brain and nervous system will respond as it is hardwired to do. When we are stressed, anxious or feel threatened in any way, our brain takes over and responds with the fight or flight response, the ancient survival mechanism. Even if we are not actually threatened, our brain and body responds as if we are. This response was discussed in the Tantra chapter in the section describing grief's impact on annamaya kosha, the physical body, and also in this chapter in the section on the yamas and brahmacharya. Practices of pratyahara can help temper the release of stress hormones and stimulate the body's relaxation response. Following are several ways to practice pratyahara that can help turn body, energy and mind inward.

- Try a detox program that can help ease the problems of fatty foods, overindulgence in alcohol or other chemicals and assist the body in feeling lighter and more able to relax.

- Take a media break. Do not watch the news or anything on TV that is upsetting or anxiety-provoking.

- Practice silence at least once a day. This can be a private time for yourself or you can share with others. No talking, listening to music or any external noise other than nature. Try longer periods of silence if possible or schedule a silent retreat.

- Turn off your cell phone, computer, tablets and televisions.

- Create your own "Moment of Zen" by focusing only on one sense very deeply. Close the eyes and focus on the sounds around you, not as separate sounds but as waves of energy. Go into your back yard or the woods and look deeply at a leaf. Eat a piece of fruit mindfully and, perhaps for the first time, truly taste.

- Choose one room and get rid of the clutter to help clear your visual and mental fields. This does not mean get rid of your beloved's belongings— you will do that when and if you are ready and if you choose. It means notice the clutter and the extra *stuff* you may have accumulated around you. Can you purge yourself, your home, your surroundings of that which you do not need?

- Practice deep relaxation, Savasana (see Hatha chapter) or progressive muscle relaxation, to go within. Use earplugs, an eye pillow and a darkened room to block out sensory input if this feels safe to you.

- Choose one yoga asana, such as Tree pose or Warrior I or II (see Hatha chapter)—and truly move into the depths of the posture. Practice it daily and search for the sense of comfort and steadiness within the pose.

Become fully present to the experience of the posture to the exclusion of all else.

❀ Practice Savasana—Corpse pose—in a quiet dark room with an eye pillow, a blanket and silence.

─────────── Experiential practice ───────────
Come to your senses

One way of calming our sensory responses is to fully come into the present moment with each of the senses, one at a time. When we have an anxiety response based on sensory (ahara) overwhelm, we can choose to move deeply into each of the senses, rather than avoid the feelings. This exercise can help you move out of an anxiety response, into sense withdrawal, more deeply into a state of concentration and, eventually, meditation.

In this exercise, you are invited to move through each of the overt physical senses, noticing and paying attention to what you are experiencing. By the end, you should notice that anxious, fearful or worrisome thoughts are lessened. Begin by taking a deep cleansing breath, roll your shoulders or your head gently, pull your shoulders up, roll them back and down, creating space between your shoulders and your ears. Take another deep breath and then begin.

First—See. Visually seeing that we are safe can help to make us feel safe. Look around your environment. What do your eyes see? You don't need to think about it, just look around the room or the space you are in and notice what you see. Name the things if you wish. *I can see my computer, I can see my salt lamp. Outside a bird drinks out of a puddle, a red car driving down the street, oak tree...* Continue with the visual scanning and noticing as long as you like, then move on to the next one.

Second—Touch. What do you feel and notice with your sense of touch? Close your eyes if it's comfortable. If not, let your gaze be soft and focused on a point about 12 inches in front of your toes. Begin with the soles of your feet and notice all the sensations you are feeling with your skin and body. Notice the pressure of the floor beneath your feet. Notice the feel of the chair against your legs, hips, bottom and back. Notice where you can feel the pressure and texture of your clothing against your skin. Do the various textures of materials feel different on different parts of your body—denim jeans compared to a lighter material of a shirt? Notice the feel and temperature of the air on your skin where it is exposed. Notice where all the parts of your body are touching and pressing against something else. Notice places on your body that are touching nothing, like the insides of your wrists or the back of your neck. Notice how your belly and chest move, rising and falling, as you breathe in and out.

Third—Listen. Bring your awareness to your sense of hearing. First bring your attention to any sounds that you become aware of outside your space. What sounds travel to your ear from beyond the door, windows or walls? Do you hear sounds far away or close by? What are they? Cars, traffic, a dog barking? Next, bring your attention to sounds inside your space. Do you hear the ticking of a clock? Your own breath? Next, bring your sense of sound within. What can you hear within your own body? Notice the sound of your own breath, moving in, moving out. Do you notice any other sounds? Can you notice the beating of your own heart, the vibration of the sound traveling through your body?

Fourth—Smell. Bring your awareness to your sense of smell. Take a deep belly breath, allowing your abdomen to expand with the breath, taking notice of the aromas you are breathing in. What can you smell? Can you smell familiar scents of your environment? A candle you were burning earlier, coffee still keeping warm, your own soap, shampoo or other toiletries? Your own personal scent? What can you smell?

Fifth—Taste. Bring your attention from your sense of smell to your sense of taste. What taste lingers on your tongue? Your double latte from this morning, toothpaste, the last thing you ate? What can you taste, if anything? Simply notice fully what taste experience you are having in this moment.

Now that all of your external senses have been attended to, rest in a space of sensory withdrawal. Notice what you feel, what you experience. When you are ready, open your eyes. If your eyes are open, look up from your downward gaze. Bring your sense of awareness back into the room and become once again present to the environment around you. If you choose, you can write about your experience in your journal. You can do this exercise anywhere, anytime. It is good for helping you to feel grounded and calm in a matter of minutes.

The sixth limb—Dharana

Dharana is concentration, fixed attention, of the mind. With this practice, the yogi moves inward. In sutra 3:1, Patanjali tells us, "Dharana is the binding of the mind to one place, object, or idea." Dharana can occur in various forms. It's what happens when a musician is focused completely on the piece she is playing, or an artist on the work he is creating. It can be seen in the athlete who is absorbed completely in the game. It is the state of flow, the "zone," concentration on one things to the exclusion of all else. We sometimes fall into this state without trying, as in the previous examples, or we can seek it out through practices of mindfulness. We can be in a state of dharana, of concentration, while holding an asana, eating a peach, gazing at a candle flame, focusing on our breath or repeating a mantra.

In grief, our ability to concentrate decreases markedly. Often referred to as "grief brain" by those in the grief community, this lack of concentration can lead to an inability to function properly on any mental task. Grief drastically impacts our cognitive processes. We may walk into a room and have no idea why we went in there. A search for lost keys can turn easily into frustration and then 20 minutes of keening and wailing after which we surprisingly find the keys in the cabinet where we keep the olives. Practicing dharana can help you to know that your brain actually does still work and can offer a space of respite for jumbled thoughts, distractedness, absent-mindedness, forgetfulness or confusion.

The practice of dharana is about fixing our concentration on something and keeping our minds focused there. When the attention wanders, as it will do, the key is to simply bring it back non-judgmentally, as many times as it takes.

It is the nature of the mind to wander. In this practice, each time you notice this has happened, bring it gently back, with compassion and love toward yourself. Remembering that our mind does so very much for us all the time. Thinking and analyzing, interpreting, remembering, wondering, questioning, searching for answers, it is only doing what it is supposed to do. This is the practice of helping the mind to be our servant, rather than the other way around.

Here are some suggestions for the practice of Dharana:

- Gazing at a flower.

- Looking at a statue or picture of your chosen deity.

- Repeating a mantra of your choice like Om, "I am Love."

- Practice gazing at a *drishti* point during asana—drishti is gazing at a fixed point in space rather than allowing the eyes to wander here and there.

- Practice *hridayakasha* dharana—*Hridaya* meaning "heart" and *akasha* meaning "space," it is a concentration and contemplation on the heart space. The Heart Light meditation in the Bhakti chapter is a good meditation to follow in order to practice hridayakasha dharana. Bring the awareness to the heart chakra space, Anahata, and allow the focus of the mind to remain.

Experiential practice
Tratak

Tratak, fixed gazing, has a profound effect on increasing concentration and aids in moving to the next step in meditation. It is a tantric practice, which seeks to awaken and move energy. Teachers also say that it helps to increase clarity of mind, strengthen the memory as well as intuitive abilities and leads to a state of heightened consciousness. It is also said to help improve eyesight and guard against diseases of the eye. For many who have difficulty with traditional meditation techniques, tratak can be very helpful, as it uses the sensory input of the eye to provide a concrete focal point that the attention can be brought back to when thoughts wander. It is also said that when a candle flame is used in tratak practice, the pineal gland can be stimulated. As the pineal is the corresponding gland of the third eye chakra, Ajna chakra, the use of a flame helps to increase intuitive ability. If you have eye problems, chronic headache or any health issues that impact the brain or pineal gland, speak to your healthcare practitioner before beginning to practice tratak.

To practice, ensure that your posture is comfortable and your lower back is supported. You may use a cushion or a chair. You may use any object you choose, such as a flower, a picture of your spiritual teacher, the deity of your choice, even a dot. I recommend practicing with a candle flame to get increased benefit to the pineal gland and because humans are drawn to the energy of the flame. When you are ready to practice, place the candle (or other object) at a comfortable distance from the eyes, not too far, not too close. Have the object at heart level or eye level, whichever feels most comfortable to your gaze. You may find it easier to practice if the background is a blank wall. Once the focal point and the seating are arranged, close the eyes and take several deep, centering breaths. You may also wish to begin with a few rounds of nadi suddhi/nadi shodhona breathing to calm the mind. Instructions for this pranayama are in the Hatha chapter (see Figures 7.72 and 7.73, pages 300-1).

To begin gazing, open the eyes and gaze at the flame. Simply gaze at the flame without taking in too much detail. The goal is to look without trying to see. Allow the eye to take in the impression of the flame without thinking about the shape or naming the colors you may see dancing in the flame. If the thoughts wander, simply acknowledge the thoughts and then allow them to float away, shifting attention fully back to the flame. Keep the eyes as steady as possible without blinking. When you feel you must blink, close the eyes gently, noticing that the impression of the flame is still visible. Release any tension from the face, mouth and jaw, take a full breath and gently open the eyes again. Tears may flow and this is okay. Resume gazing.

When practicing tratak, you may feel that your energy is separate from your body. You may see colors or spots, you may feel light or you may feel movement of prana in different areas of the body. Do not be alarmed if you notice any of these things, they often occur naturally in energy practices. Always close the eyes if gazing becomes uncomfortable, take a breath, release tension and then resume gently gazing. A beginning tratak practice should be about 5 to 10 minutes. You might increase the time by a few minutes each practice session until you reach 30 or 40 minutes if you wish.

The seventh limb—Dhyana

Dhyana, meditation, is the seventh limb of Raja. Dharana, the sixth limb, prepares the mind by sharpening focus for the state of dhyana. Legendary teacher B.K.S. Iyengar wrote in *The Tree of Yoga* (1988), "Focusing on one point is concentration. Focusing on all points at the same time is meditation… Concentration has a point of focus; meditation has no points. That is the secret" (p.41-42). Most of the time, when we sit to meditate, what we are really practicing is dharana, concentration.

When we are truly in a state of meditation, we are unaware of time passing. In the state of dharana, when we are still concentrating rather than meditating, we may wonder when the timer will sound, how long we have been sitting, bringing our thoughts back to the anchor, over and over. In a state of meditation, we do none of those things, we are absorbed. As Inyengar also taught, meditation is integration. When we conceive or think in any way that our body, mind and spirit are separate, the true state of meditation shows us that this is not true. In dhyana, we are reintegrated.

In dharana, concentration, we become distracted; thoughts rise and we are distracted from our focus. We refocus and there is restraint of thought, then another thought may come. In the space between those thoughts is a moment of tranquility, of passivity. With practice, that moment, the space between, comes more easily and stays longer. That space is dhyana, meditation; a space of no thought, a sense of spaciousness, a merging into Oneness—with all aspects of self as well as with the entire Universe. If we can come to that space of Oneness with ourselves, our beloved dead can be part of that space also. Without thought, without questioning, without the continual seeking and searching that are all part of the activity of the mind, the ego and its constant need to be separate, we can rest in a space where past and future drop away. It is an experience that cannot truly be described because it occurs in a space of no words. It is a space of non-duality and we cannot speak about non-duality without duality. It is a space of peace.

In grief, peace can be hard to find. Meditation can help us reach that space where we can have peace in the midst of the pain and perhaps find a way of connecting with our loved ones as well. As we know, grief ravages the body, mind and spirit. A great deal of research has been done in the past two decades on the benefits of meditation and mindfulness practices. Meditation-based techniques such as Mindfulness-Based Stress Reduction (MBSR), based on the work of John Kabat-Zinn, and Mindfulness-Based Cognitive Therapies (MBCT) have much research to support the immense and far reaching benefits of the practice. Study after study shows that anxiety, depression, eating disorders, substance abuse, anger problems and insomnia can be effectively treated with meditation mindfulness strategies. Other studies have shown increased immune function, the ability to have better focus and attention, reduction in experiences associated with traumatic stress including hypervigilance and hyperarousal, and an increased sense of calm even when we are not in meditation. The benefits are pervasive and cumulative. With meditation we can find relief from the immense stress of grief; a space of respite from the constant jumble of thoughts, the doubt, painful self-talk, incessant questioning, feelings of anger, deprivation, sadness, hopelessness, fear, longing, yearning; and a sense of deep connectedness with All.

If we can realize that the boundaries and separations that we perceive in ourselves are false, that they do not exist, we can become aware that there is no separation among anyone or anything. Body, mind, spirit, soul, are one. If this is true for us, then it is also true for our beloved dead. As above, so below, as within, so without. We can never be separate. The self that we think we know, the "I" and "me" that is the center of our own known universe dissolves in that state of awareness. We can feel a very real sense of unity with those we love who have died. It is not possible to feel alone or unloved in that state. There we know that we are at One with everything and everyone. This is whole, that is whole. When a portion of wholeness is removed, what remains is whole. Entering this space of wholeness is rest and peace.

Mindful meditation

This is a version of Vipassana meditation, an ancient Indian practice which means insight, "to see things as they really are."

I suggest starting with a goal of five minutes a day and work up slowly, adding a minute on to your time weekly. If five seems like too much, start with three or four. Use a timer so that you don't feel compelled to check the clock. Turn off your phone and other technological devices that could interrupt you. Find a comfortable spot. You can sit in a chair or on the floor. If you sit on the floor, use a cushion or meditation bench to sit on so that your hips are higher than your knees. If you choose to sit in a chair, let your feet be flat on the floor. Allow your hands to rest in your lap or on your knees in a comfortable position. If you wish, take jnana mudra (see Figure 2.2, page 36) if it will not be a distraction from the practice. Allow your spine to be long and tall, but not stiff. Roll your neck from side to side to release tension. Take a few deep, cleansing breaths deep into your belly. Allow your breathing to return to normal.

Then, simply begin to notice. Notice how the floor feels beneath your feet. Notice the feeling of your body at the points where it rests either on the floor or against the chair, how your clothes feel on your body. Notice the feeling of the material of your clothing against your skin. Notice whether you feel any tension in any area of your body. Simply notice. Begin to notice the temperature of the air, notice how it feels on the parts of your body that are uncovered. You don't have to do anything to change, just notice. Begin to notice the sounds that you hear around you; in the room, outside the room. Note any sounds you may become aware of within your own body. Bring your awareness to your breath. Notice how it feels as it moves in and out of your body. Allow your attention to remain with your breath, in and out, notice the temperature of the air as it enters your nose, moves down your trachea and into your lungs. Notice that it is warmer and more moist as it gently leaves your body. Notice the movements of your abdomen, your ribs and your chest as your breath moves in and out of your body.

Continue to simply stay with your breath. If you wish, you can count your breaths, in and out, 1, in and out 2, and so on to 10 and then return to 1. You might want to use color visualizations with your breath—breathing in a color you associate with a feeling state you would like to achieve, such as peace or calm, then breathing out a color you associate with a feeling you would like to be rid of such as fear, stress, anxiety, or pain. You might want to use a mantra with your in/out breaths. On an in breath, think, "I am..." and on an out breath, "calm."

Come up with whatever works for you to help you stay with your breath. Eventually, you will notice you are no longer aware of your breath and instead, you are thinking about something else. This is ok, and it will happen, this is what the mind does. When you notice that you're thinking or an emotion rises, simply label it and gently bring your focus back to your breath.

Label your thoughts and emotions: thinking, worrying, planning, doubting, judging, fantasizing, anxiety, fear, impatience, irritation. Then bring your attention back to your breath. "Thinking"...come back to the breath... "Planning"...come back to the breath... "Anxiety"...come back to the breath... "Judging"...come back to the breath. If you are distracted by a sound, label it—"birds," "car," "people outside"—and come back to the breath. The returning and returning to the breath is dharana, concentration. Continue in this way until your time is completed for the day's practice. After your timer goes off, take a moment to notice how you are feeling. Take a couple of deep breaths and go on with your day. You will notice the more you practice, the faster the time goes by and the longer the spaces between thoughts and feelings that rise. The space between is dhyana. Meditation.

The eighth limb—Samadhi

Rather like anandamaya kosha, the sheath of pure bliss beyond which our True Self is found, there is little to say about samadhi. Samadhi is the final limb in Patanjali's Raja yoga. Swami Satchidananda says this, "Meditation culminates in the state of samadhi. It's not that you practice samadhi. Nobody can consciously practice samadhi" (p.175). Samadhi is the ultimate Union; the state which results from the practice of all the previous limbs. It is the space in which all separation falls away, yet full consciousness remains. A super-consciousness is attained when the conscious, subconscious and the unconscious aspects of our minds are united. All the koshas are experienced as one fluid Self, joined also with the Universal Consciousness, Oneness. All levels of reality are merged.

From the space of samadhi, which is a space and state that includes all states, comes enlightenment, revelation of all truth and what Patanjali calls the *siddhis*, or accomplishments. There are various levels of samadhi, but for our purposes, there are two basic levels. One in which we experience the Oneness with All, which could be compared with the bliss of the moment, wherein even the smallest degree of samadhi can help increase inner peace and release the force of repeating Karmic patterns that may be creating pain mentally, physically and energetically. The other type of samadhi is a more permanent samadhi in which a state of super-consciousness, bliss and realization of Oneness is permanently maintained, yet we are able to go about our lives performing normal human functions. Whether we reach that level of samadhi is not relevant, striving to reach it will not get us there, but rather the ongoing increasing amount of peace, harmony and steadiness of mind that the practices of yoga can bring.

Chapter 7

Hatha Yoga

The Path of Sun and Moon

Hatha Yoga is generally considered to be any yoga that has to do with the physical body. All teachers agree that this includes asana, the postures, and pranayama, breathing techniques. Some include pratyahara (sense withdrawal), dharana (concentration), dhyana (meditation), as well as chant and some of the *kriyas*, internal actions that include certain cleansing processes. Hatha in all its aspects is meant to bring balance, harmony, sattva to the first three koshas. Balance in body, mind and energy.

The word Hatha itself is balance. In Sanskrit, *ha* means "sun" and *tha* means "moon." Hatha represents the balance of warmth and coolness, conscious and subconscious, masculine and feminine, body with mind. It is a method by which we can find the balance sufficient to move toward meditation and spiritual wholeness. Each asana is also about the balance of sun and moon, heat and cool. Renowned teacher B.K.S. Iyengar taught that every posture requires two things: a sense of direction and a sense of one's center of gravity. The word asana itself tells us we must have a balance between steady and comfortable. Finding that balance is Hatha yoga.

This chapter delves into several asana chosen for their energetic effects on the koshas and describes ways that each particular asana is helpful in grief. The chapter also suggests several pranayama practices that will help calm the body and mind, energize and detoxify. Mantra and chant practices are also shared. Before practicing any aspects of Hatha yoga, please discuss with your health care practitioner your fitness and ability to engage in yoga practices. Some postures are contraindicated for some particular health issues and these will be addressed. Always use caution and good sense and take care to ensure safety.

Yoga asana

The second edition of the text *Yoga Anatomy* (Kaminoff and Matthews 2012) tells us that each pose is "a container for an experience." Executing each pose, "we experience a cross section of a never-ending progression of movement and breath, extending infinitely forward and backward in time" (p.65). In every posture, we are given the opportunity to experience fully what our container communicates, feels, holds, releases and bears. Each asana also gives us the opportunity to sink deeply as well as to transcend. The yin and yang, stillness and movement, of energy help us recognize and learn to work with, cope and manage the varied states of being we experience at any given time.

The essential obvious feature which separates yoga asana from other form of bodily exercise and movement is the focus on the breath and the mindfulness of movement combined with the breath. Generally, we exhale with any contraction and inhale as we expand. We use the breath to help us deepen postures, as a focal point, to energize as well as to relax body and mind. Yoga teaches us to be present to what is, to accept where we are right now, in the present. It teaches us to adjust as we need to in order to be comfortable yet steady; to adapt and accommodate in order to maintain our comfortable steady posture, not only in asana or on the yoga mat, but in our daily lives.

Understand that the postures of yoga are not simply physical movements or poses we twist, turn or fold our bodies into. They are, according to yogic science, philosophy and tradition, divinely inspired. Because of this, asana benefits the body greatly, but also affects the other koshas as well. We experience the effects of each pose in the physical body, the energy and mental bodies, intellectually, emotionally and on deep levels of intuition and beyond. Many yoga postures will feel good, and many will create some discomfort not only bodily, but mentally and emotionally. *This does not mean pain in the body.* If any asana creates or exacerbates pain in the body, *do not do it.* The postures are designed to help us deepen into full experiences as humans and spiritual beings; injury is not a requirement for full experience of asana.

Often the postures that are the most difficult emotionally are the ones we need to explore the most. Each posture stimulates and works with the energy as well as the samskaras—Karmic patterns—of each yogi. Intense emotional release can occur in any posture. Sometimes these experiences may feel overwhelming, particularly if they are unexpected. These occurrences, including physical and the emotional releases help move us to a more sattvic state of balance and harmony—within and without. Allowing ourselves to release in a pose can help break through potentially years of holding and struggling and resisting. The more we hold the pain that does not serve us, the more we are likely to repeat patterns of behavior and thinking that keep us from experiencing the balance that is our natural state of being. The practices of yoga, including asana, help us to consciously and compassionately release and clear obstacles to our wholeness.

The postures

For all of the asana offered here, the Sanskrit is given as well as the English.

Yogic eye movements—Netra vyayamam

netra=eyes *vyayamam*=exercise, movement

The eye movements help to relieve eye fatigue, strain and soreness that can come from crying, reading, rubbing, straining, squinting and staring at screens including phones, tablets, televisions and computers. We often do not realize how much work our eyes do for us and how much rest they require. Our eyes may be the most overused and abused of all the sense organs.

Netra vyayamam can help ease the strain we constantly place on our eyes. Due to increased tension in the muscles of the face, neck and head area, the ocular nerves and muscles surrounding the eyes of grieving people can be far more stressed and overworked than the eyes of non-grieving people. Irritation, redness and swelling of the delicate tissues around the eyes resulting from lack of sleep, excessive crying and rubbing, all contribute to fatigue, pain, and strain of the eyes. The eyes of a grieving person are stressed beyond belief. They need rest.

In addition to relief of physical tension, bilateral eye movements engaging both sides of the brain may help to balance the hemispheres of the brain which when chronically flooded with cortisol and other stress hormones can result in problems with focus, cognition, attention, working memory and self-regulation. Yogic eye movements allow the eyes to find relief and rest as well as serving to tone the ocular nerves and the muscles of the eyes. Traditionally, yogis teach that eye movements improve vision over time, extend years of good vision and can even potentially remove disease from the eyes.

The eye movements also work to increase our inner visionary abilities. The sages tell us that netra vyayamam can potentially result in development of clairvoyant abilities and the attainment of deep spiritual insight and revelation. For yogis, the outer sense of sight is intimately attached to inner sight. Visualization of any kind requires the use of our inner sight, the ability to imagine and "see" things that are not physically present, as well as insight, intuitive or deep understanding. In the yogic way of thinking, there is no separation: The physical sight, inner sight and insight are joined.

To practice the eye movements (Figure 7.1, page 229), find a comfortable seated position, either on the floor or on a chair. Allow the spine to be long, but not stiff. Remove glasses or hard contact lenses. In the eye movements, move the eyes only, and not the head or neck. When you are ready, begin with the vertical movement, looking upward as far as is comfortable. Raise the eyebrows if that is comfortable for you. Hold here for 20 to 30 seconds. Then, with the eyebrows relaxed, direct the gaze downward as far as is comfortable for you. Again hold for 20 to 30 seconds. Close the eyes and allow them to relax. When you are ready, open the eyes and look to the right as far as is comfortable for you. Hold for 20 to 30 seconds. Then move the gaze as far as possible to the left. Hold again 20 to 30 seconds. Close the eyes. Notice how the eyes feel. Take a breath and relax the eyes.

Next, you'll gradually move the eyes in a circle. It may help to imagine a large clock face with numbers in front of you. Open the eyes and look as far upward as is comfortable to the 12 o'clock point on the clock. Allow them to move to each point on the clock face, 1, 2, 3, 4 o'clock, and so on around the clock until you reach 12 once more. If you find that your eyes skip a point on the clock, go back to the point you skipped and begin again at that point. At each point on the clock face, you are stretching the eyes and taking the gaze as far to the perimeter as possible while remaining comfortable. When you reach the 12 o'clock point close the eyes and relax. Open the eyes and move the eyes counter-clockwise from 12 o'clock, to 11, to 10 and so on. When you reach 12 in the counter-clockwise movements, close the eyes once more.

Opening the eyes, continue to imagine the large clock face. For the next set of exercises, you will move the eyes once again around the clock face, but rather than touching on each individual point on the clock, allow the gaze to sweep smoothly around the circle with continuous movement. Again, if you find that your eyes skip over any point, simply go back and resume the smooth movement from there. Allow the eyes to move clockwise in a circle, at the farthest edge of your vision, once or twice if you are comfortable. When you reach the 12 o'clock point on the clock, stop and close the eyes, allowing them to rest. When you are ready, open the eyes and bring the gaze again to 12 o'clock and begin the same circular movement in a counter-clockwise direction. Go slowly and do not rush. Allow the gaze to move around the circle once or twice. When you reach 12, close the eyes and relax the gaze.

With the eyes closed, bring the palms of the hands together and rub them together briskly until you create heat in the center of your palms. Cup your hands over the eyes and allow the eyes to bathe in the warmth and darkness of the palms. Imagine the warmth and energy from the palms sinking into the eyes. As the eyes relax, send a message of thanks to your eyes for all the work they do for you. When the heat of the palms dissipates, lightly brush the brows and lids with the fingertips, stroking outward and upward with gentle movements. If you like, from here you may wish to massage the forehead, temples, the jaw and back of the neck.

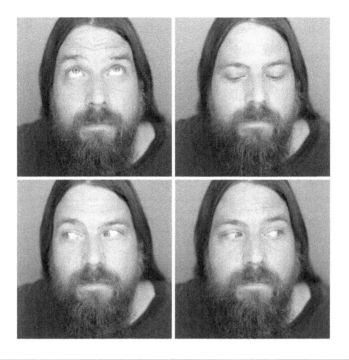

Figure 7.1 The eye movements.

Sun salutation—Surya namaskar

surya=sun *namaskar*=to bow, to adore

Surya namaskar, a flowing series of asana combining movement of the body with inhalation and exhalation as the body expands and contracts, is a common sequence seen in many yoga classes. Traditionally, surya namaskar is not just a series of bodily movements, it is a prayer, an offering to Lord Surya, god of the sun and of health. The sun is also seen as the physical and spiritual heart of the world, the most vital source of energy, bringing light, heat and allowing growth. It is helpful to perform surya namaskar every day to establish a ritual that can empower body, mind and spirit.

Energizing and strengthening, surya namaskar increases flexibility and circulation. The series of postures can benefit the entire body, promoting spine flexibility and loosening each joint. The muscles of the abdomen, the back, the arms, legs and pelvis are toned and strengthened. Done slowly, the movements can have a calming, meditative effect and when done more rapidly, can invigorate, energize and create heat in the body. Emotionally, sun salute can help to counteract feelings of depletion, disconnection and sadness. By connecting with the energy of the sun, our source of warmth and growth, tapas, we can feel more connected to and part of the world around us. Done with full mindfulness and intention, sun salute can be offered as a moving meditation or prayer which can transform and ease the pain of grief and loss. You may stay in any of the postures as long as you wish, paying attention to the flow of the breath, inhaling as you expand, exhaling as you fold or contract.

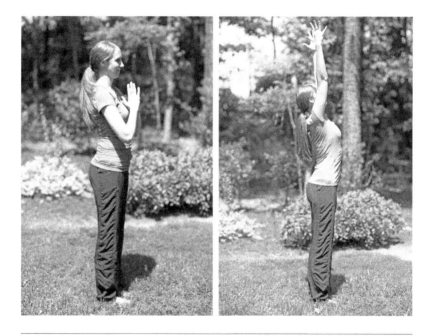

Figure 7.2 (1) Begin with anjali mudra standing in *tadasana*, the mountain pose (see next asana).

Figure 7.3 (2) Inhale, reaching upward with a micro backbend, keeping the knees soft to protect the lower back.

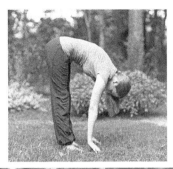

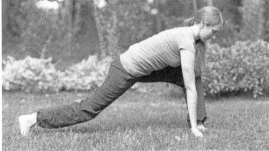

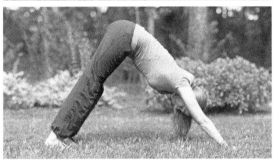

Figure 7.4 (3) Exhale folding forward from the hips into *uttanasana*, forward fold, keeping the spine long, reaching the heart forward. When you come to your maximum fold, remember to keep the posture steady and comfortable, allow the head, neck, and arms to relax. Pause and notice the breath moving in and out of the body. With each exhalation, allow the body to fold a little more.

Figure 7.5 (4) Bring the fingers to the mat, inhale and step the right leg back as far as is comfortable into a lunge. You can choose to bring the knee to the floor or keep it raised. Allow the hips to sink toward the floor. Make sure the left knee doesn't extend outward over the toes. You may wish to stay here a few breaths.

Figure 7.6 (5) Exhale, taking the left leg back to meet the right into downward facing dog. Keep the knees bent if this is more comfortable. You may wish to pedal the heels, alternately stretching the calves as is comfortable. To find the correct spinal alignment, come up on your toes and tilt the sit bones upward, as if you were going to sit on the ceiling, then gently release the heels toward the floor. Pedal the heels, gently stretching the calf muscles if you wish.

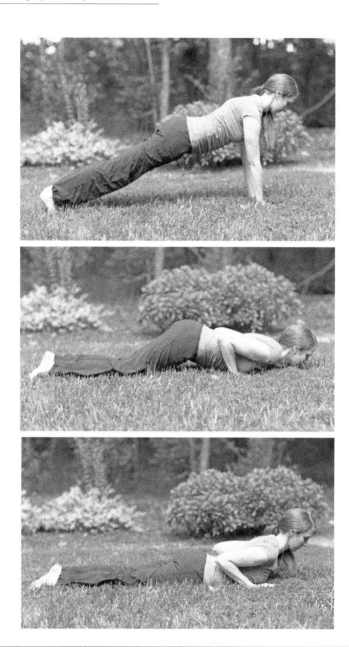

Figure 7.7 (6) Inhale, and moving the heart forward, come into a plank position.
Keep the core strong, not allowing the hips to dip toward the floor. If plank
is not possible or comfortable, come to hands and knees (see Figure 7.16).
Feel free to do cat/cow movement here if you wish (see Figures 7.17–18).

Figure 7.8 (7) Exhale, bringing the knees, chest, chin to the mat.

Figure 7.9 (8) Inhale, move forward into cobra pose, hands beneath
the shoulders, elbows close to the body and pointing upward, squeeze
the shoulder blades together, lift the chest and gaze forward.

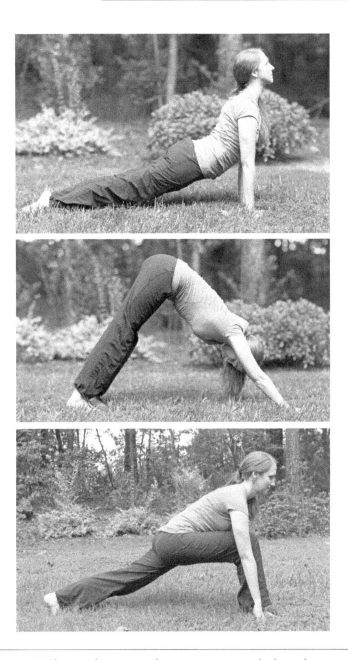

Figure 7.10 (9) If you wish, you may choose to come into a higher cobra or upward facing dog. Press the tops of the feet into the mat, lifting the chest, hips and thighs off the mat. Check that the shoulders are not hunched up toward the ears.

Figure 7.11 (10) Exhaling again, lift the hips upward and come again into downward facing dog.

Figure 7.12 (11) Inhale, bring the right leg forward between the hands into the second lunge, again allowing the hips to drop toward the floor. Check that your right knee is not extending beyond the big toe. Allow the hips to release downward.

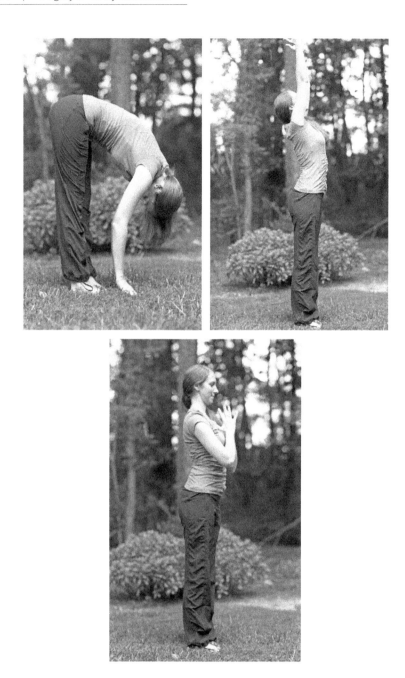

Figure 7.13 (12) Bring the left foot to meet the right
foot, exhale back to uttanasana, forward fold.

Figure 7.14 (13) Inhale, keeping the knees soft, reach the
arms overhead, with a micro backbend if you wish.

Figure 7.15 (14) Exhale and bring hands to the heart in anjali mudra,
returning to the beginning pose, tadasana, mountain pose.

Mountain Pose—Tadasana

tada=mountain

This standing posture energizes the whole body. In it, you practice complete stillness and full activity of major muscle groups while opening your heart, focusing on breathing and strengthening your whole body. You can do this pose anywhere, anytime. See Figure 7.2 in the sun salutation series for a photo of tadasana.

When taking tadasana, bring the arms alongside the body first to feel balanced fully on both feet. Have the feet together or hip width apart, whatever feels steadier. Rock slightly from the balls of the feet to the heels, finding balance. Allow the weight to be evenly distributed on both feet. Let the knees be straight, soft, not locked. The hips should be directly over the ankles. Lengthen the spine upward, roll the shoulders up, back and down, releasing them away from the ears. Extend the back of the neck upward, tucking the chin slightly. Leave the arms down, hands relaxed, fingers pointing toward the Earth, or spread the palms wide. You may turn the palms toward the thighs or rotate the wrists so the palms face out, or bring the hands together at the heart into anjali mudra. Do what feels good to you. Feel as though you are aligning the energies of your body in the way that is right for you, right now. Feel your feet grounded into the Earth, your feet like the base of a mountain, strong, steady and rooted. Imagine your head reaching upward into the sky like a mountain peak. Feel your chest expand and open, receiving the rays of the sun. Breathe.

Cat/Cow—Marjariasana/Bitilasana

marjari=cat *bitil*=cow

This combination of postures strengthens and relaxes the spine. This movement, coordinated with the breath, can be very helpful at bedtime, encouraging the release of tension in the spine, neck and lower back. Moving with the breath helps us to be more aware of the breath, deepening each inhale and exhale, allowing a calming effect on the mind. Emotionally and energetically, cat/cow movement can be very powerful.

Though it is a simple movement, it stimulates all the chakras and facilitates the flow of energy throughout the spine and sushumna, the major nadi which corresponds with the spinal cord. Expanding and contracting, the flow moves us from passive to active energy, sending energy outward and holding it in. Cat/cow can soothe tension and anxiety and help to release fears and insecurities stored in Muladhara, the root chakra. The movement of the pelvic space can also work to discharge residual or stuck energies from emotional distress stored within Svadisthana, the sacral chakra. It can help us feel our own power in Manipura the solar plexus, while expanding Anahata, the heart chakra, and Vishuddha, the throat chakra, from the front as well as the back. Ajna, the third eye, and Sushumna, the crown chakra, are gently soothed as well. As you move the body, be mindful of sensations, images or feelings that may arise.

To practice cat/cow, come to hands and knees in table top position with a neutral spine, looking downward at the floor between your hands (Figure 7.16). Wrists beneath elbows, elbows beneath shoulders, knees hip width apart. Stabilize the shoulder blades by drawing them gently down the back. Inhaling, simultaneously left the head, allow the belly to drop toward the floor, the chest to move forward, the shoulders to move away from the ears, and the sitting bones to reach toward the ceiling, creating the silhouette of a swayback cow (Figure 7.17). As you exhale, drop the head toward the floor, slightly tucking the chin (without force), tuck the tailbone, draw the pubic bone forward, while arching the spine upward toward the ceiling creating the line of an arched back cat (Figure 7.18). Continue this movement with your own easeful breath. You may also wish to incorporate a gentle c-curve movement of the spine from the table top position. Inhale at neutral spine, exhale and bring the head toward the right hip, looking backward at the right foot. Inhale to neutral, exhale bringing the head toward the left hip, looking back toward the left foot, continue using the flow of your own breath.

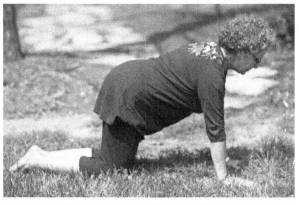

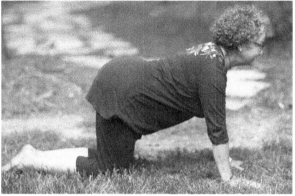

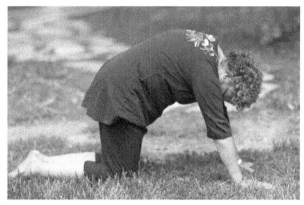

Figure 7.16 (1) Table top pose, neutral spine.

Figure 7.17 (2) Cow, inhaling.

Figure 7.18 (3) Cat, exhaling.

Kali asana—Utkata konasana

utkata=fierce *kona*=angle

This pose is often referred to as Goddess pose as well as Victory Squat. I call it Kali asana, because it reminds me of the powerful Goddess Kali whose fierce sword can cut away all that which no longer serves us.

All of Hatha yoga, and therefore all asana, grew from Tantric traditions of honoring and revering everything manifest in the physical world as the expression of Shakti, the primal feminine force of all creation. Most asana are modeled after things in the natural world, animals, shapes, various elements of all creation, which we mirror by taking the form of those things in a formal posture with our bodies. In this way, we are honoring all creation around us as well as our own bodies.

The Goddess pose represents the direct power of the Mother's creation. No one should mistake it as a pose meant only for women. Men, in grief and in life, are also in need of connecting to the power of the Great Mother. Both men and women hold yin and yang energies that serve to create balance within and without. The power of the feminine is overlooked and undermined, repressed and dismissed, for women in the yang, or active expression and for men in the yin, or passive expression. This can be problematic for both sexes.

For men, the "strong, silent type" may be seen as desirable at some point, but if he chooses not to act by asserting overt, typically "masculine" power, he may be belittled and dismissed. A woman who asserts her yang power of creation and control may be called bossy or bitchy, and is often pushed and pressured to resume the more socially acceptable yin role of passive nurturing and submissive deference.

While the yang energy of a man is typically and widely accepted as outwardly directed, dominating, with external action, the feminine yang energy is centered and grows from within; think of the explosive, unstoppable power that is physical birth. That force of birth begins from within and is ultimately transformative, changing not only the world around us, but ourselves from within. A man's yin energy is that of patience, storing up of power which can find expression in many forms, not just the aggressive, dominant form that is typically expected. A man can be soft, nurturing, loving and tender, just as a woman can be strong, fierce, direct and powerful. The Goddess nurtures these qualities.

Like so many things it touches, grief can break the masculine/feminine stereotypes to pieces. Both men and women in grief and bereavement search for ways to express the pain and sorrow of grief. We can all be transformed by its power. The imagery of the Goddess is a perfect vehicle for this kind of expression. Men are often overlooked in their grief and disallowed full expression of their experiences. This can result in painful and sometimes disastrous outcomes. Grief not allowed expression can result in further isolation, denial or repression of feelings, resulting in withdrawal from emotional experiences or intimacy with others, increased potential to medicate the experience of grief through substance overuse or abuse, an imbalance of anger resulting in abusive or destructive behavior toward self and others.

This can happen to both men and women; neither love nor grief is solely a masculine or feminine, male or female, experience. Each person grieves individually. Our society, however, has particular expectations of how a man or a woman is "supposed" to grieve. Or to love. Or to heal. Women can find more, though still limited, acceptance in outward expression of tears and other visible signs of grief as well as permission for more vocal communication about feelings and experiences. For men this is rare. When any of us feel forced to fit into a certain category, to deny our experience, to "get over it," to "man up," to "move on" or any other clichéd supposition, our own process of integrating experiences of loss into who we are as full beings is blocked.

The Goddess is our Mother. In grief and life, the energy, support and love of a Mother is all. Without Her we could not survive. With Her, we are nurtured, empowered, lifted up and above all loved beyond measure. Practices of Tantra and of asana in general can serve to help both men and women to balance and more fully embrace the yin and the yang of the Mother within.

You are invited as you practice this asana to fully embody the energy of the Mother, in her power and creativity, her strength and her love.

This version of Kali asana is inspired by Sally Kempton's *Awakening Shakti* (2013) and can stir the power of Kali Ma in your life. The fierce Goddess Kali is the ultimate representation of the ability to hold both light and dark simultaneously. In her ferocity She is absolute wildness. She represents abandon of social rules and constructs. She is fearsome and liberating at the same time. She is the body of the Universe which holds birth and death and everything in between, shattering obstacles and removing limitations. She can hold us up in the midst of all manner of destruction.

Psychotherapist Francis Weller, in his work *Entering the Healing Ground* (2012), writes, "There is something feral about grief, something essentially outside the ordained and sanctioned behaviors of our culture… Grief is alive, wild, untamed and cannot be domesticated. It resists the demands to remain passive and still" (p.8). This is an apt metaphor for both the wild, primal force of grief and the energy of Kali. Anyone who has experienced the ancient keening moans and guttural cries of unfathomable loss has touched the power of Kali. Embracing Her power as part of ourselves allows us to move beyond the fear of grief and into the freedom that can come with abandonment of all that is extraneous and false.

To practice, begin with the feet a bit wider than hip width apart, feet turned out slightly so the knees can bend easily (Figure 7.19). Inhaling, send the arms overhead, palms and fingers spread (Figure 7.19). Exhale as you deeply bend the knees while bringing the elbows downward so the biceps are at shoulder height. Fingers splayed, feet rooted, thighs, arms and back strong, open the mouth, stick out your tongue and from your belly, rather than your throat, shout, "AHHH!!" (Figure 7.20). Bring the shout from the belly rather from the throat. Inhale back to standing, bringing the arms over the head once more. Repeat the movement three to five times. Notice how you feel afterward.

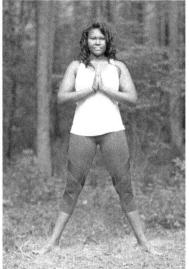
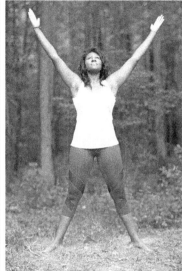

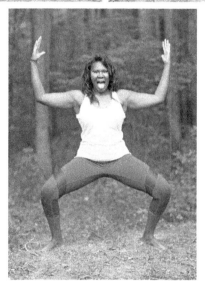

Figure 7.19 (1) Begin in anjali mudra, feet wide, so the knees can bend comfortably.

Figure 7.20 (2) Bring the hands and arms overhead, reaching
upward to the sky, look upward if this feels right to you.

Figure 7.21 (3) Bend the knees, pulling the elbows
downward, sticking out your tongue in Kali asana.

Backbends

All backbending postures increase flexibility and strengthen the back as well as create dynamic energy. They open and expand the chest wall as well as the heart chakra. In backbending postures particularly, our heart and throat chakras are wide open and front facing. Both of these are also accessible from the back, but when we backbend, the energy we express is fully open at our front bodies and moving outward into the world: We are fully exposed. This can be a vulnerable space for those in grief. Because of this please be aware that backbending asana can create strong emotional responses in the heart, belly or throat spaces.

What we do to and with the body, we also do to and with the mind and spirit. When our energetic bodies have been closed or hurt, and then those areas are opened, we can experience emotional, energetic and even physical discomfort. How we think about this discomfort makes all the difference. If we are unprepared, if we do not know that these physical postures can result in these kinds of reactions, we can be afraid, taken by surprise, and want to shut down the pain, to stop the hurting. We may feel embarrassed, confused or unsafe. Knowing ahead of time that actions we take with the physical body (annamayakosha) impacts all other layers of our being, we can be prepared. We can even plan for and welcome the process as an opportunity for growth and expression.

Often when I speak about the expression of grief and other painful emotions and experiences, I explain "expression" in terms of not just sharing or making known one's thoughts or feelings, but the act of physical expressing, of squeezing, pressing, removing something.

Yoga asana and the effects on the mind, body and spirit can be seen in this way. Trauma and pain are stored in every cell of our bodies. Asana is a practice that can manipulate the gross and subtle bodies in ways that facilitate expression and release. Physical toxins can be released from tissues, emotional and spiritual pain can be allowed discharge. Space can be created for new growth, new experience, new love and healing, where healing is needed, can occur. During asana practice it is not unusual to experience the urge to cry or to laugh or to experience other spontaneous outpourings of emotional expression. Please do not be surprised to experience intense emotion during asana practices. And know that this is okay. You can be safe and loved, even in feelings of uncertainty.

Cobra—Bhujangasana

bhujang=cobra

Bhujangasana can help facilitate strength of self and a sense of openness toward others and the world. It is a posture of giving and receiving without judgment. The heart and the throat chakras are opened in this posture. If you have felt unable to fully communicate or express your thoughts and feelings, if your voice has been shut down or cut off, if your heart has felt closed or closely protected, emotional and energetic pain may be released in this posture. Bhujangasana cultivates courage and determination and helps ease worry. Physically, the posture helps to develop flexibility in the upper spine, stretches and strengthens the muscles of the neck and back, tones the abdominal organs and increases circulation around the spine.

To come into cobra, lie on the belly, with the forehead to the mat, palms down, directly under the shoulders. The elbows should be close to the body (Figure 7.22). Gently, as if you are rolling a marble with your nose, stretch the chin forward, slowly raising the head, neck and chest, rolling the vertebrae back. Squeeze the shoulder blades together to increase the awareness there, noticing the energy in the chest and throat. Keep the neck extended, taking care not to compress the vertebrae. Lift the hands slightly to ensure that you are using the muscles of the back and not the arms (Figure 7.23). To release the posture, slowly bring the forehead back down to the mat.

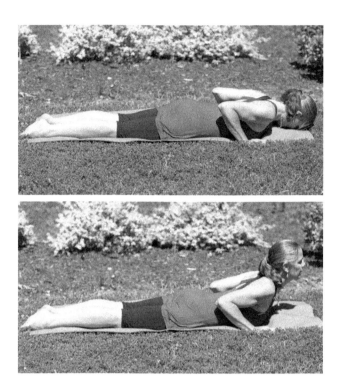

Figure 7.22 (1) Preparation for bhujangasana.

Figure 7.23 (2) Full posture.

Bow pose and half bow pose—Dhanurasana and ardha dhanurasana

dhanu=bow *ardha*=half

Bow pose can help us to feel our own internal strength. Opening the chest, it helps balance Anahata, the heart chakra, and Svadisthana, the sacral chakra. Deep emotional pain can be held in the sacral chakra. Remnants of pain and grief from relationships and childhood trauma is also held in this space. The sacral chakra is connected with the water element and, in dhanurasana, the body can be allowed to gently rock with the breath, creating a gentle, wavelike motion, soothing the energy of this space. Bow pose is associated with helping to free creative expression and increases our ability to release any sense of responsibility toward others that is unwarranted.

Both full and half bow poses extend the entire spine, stretch the pectoral muscles and the hip area. Half bow pose done from a hands and knees position is also a good balancing pose (Figures 7.24–25). When doing half bow, always balance out by doing both sides. If half bow is done from the abdomen, bring the forearm forward under the chest to help stabilize the posture.

To prepare for dhanurasana, lie on the abdomen, bend the knees, bringing the heels toward your buttocks. Take hold of the ankles with the hands. Bring the forehead to the mat (Figure 7.26). You may remain in the preparatory pose as long as you like. To come into your bow, press the legs into the hands, lift the lower half of the body and then arch the head, neck and chest upward. Relax the shoulders back and look upward (Figure 7.27). Breathe. Go into child's pose, *balasana* (Figure 7.70), as a counter posture.

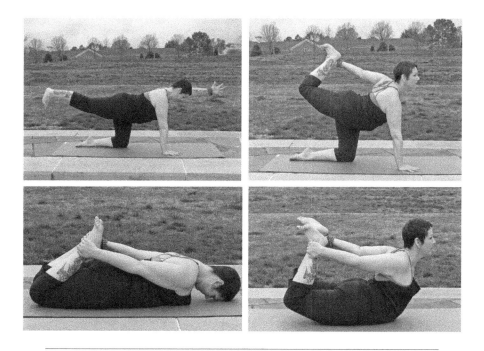

Figure 7.24 (1) From table top position, practice spinal balance.

Figure 7.25 (2) Half bow.

Figure 7.26 (3) Grasp ankles.

Figure 7.27 (4) Press ankles into hands, full bow pose.

Wheel pose—Chakrasana or upward facing bow pose—Urdhva dhanurasana

urdhva=upward *dhanu*=bow *chakra*=wheel

Wheel pose helps to open the entire chest and stimulates the thyroid and the pituitary glands, helping to relieve feelings of sadness. It is a dynamic posture that increases hip and spine flexibility and energizes the respiratory system. If you have a back injury, carpal tunnel syndrome, digestive problems, shoulder problems, heart problems, high or low blood pressure, please avoid this posture.

To come into wheel, lie on the floor on your back. Bend the knees and place your feet flat on the floor. Bring the heels as close to the sitting bones as possible. Bend the elbows and spread your palms on the floor beside the head, fingers pointing toward your shoulders. Press the feet into the floor, exhale, and push the tailbone upward, lifting the hips off the floor. Stay here if you like. To come into full wheel, press the hands into the floor and lift up gently onto the crown of the head. Pressing the hands and feet into the floor, lift the head off the floor and straighten your arms. Keep the thighs firm and continue lifting the hips upward. Allow the head to hang (Figure 7.28). Stay in the pose for only as long as is comfortable, up to three minutes. To come out of the pose, bend the arms and legs, tuck the chin into the chest and gently lower the spine to the floor. As a counter pose after wheel, take child's pose (Figure 7.70), or lie on your back bringing your knees into your chest, to rock gently.

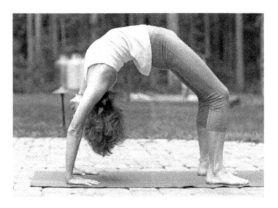

Figure 7.28 (2) Full chakrasana.

Camel pose—Ustrasana

ustra=camel

Camel pose is a stretch of the entire front of the body and a deep backbend, which opens the heart space fully. Camel pose in particular can open and create a release of painful feelings stored in the chest and heart area. Extreme emotional responses are not uncommon in camel pose, including sobbing or laughter. This posture can cause us to feel extremely open and vulnerable. If you experience emotions in this posture, try to simply witness the emotions or thoughts as they come with as much compassion as possible. Ustrasana can help balance the chakras, particularly the heart and throat chakras, but works on the entire chakra system. Physically, it opens hips and helps to ease tension in the ovaries. It stretches the ankles, thighs, groin, abdomen, chest and throat, improves flexibility in the spine and helps with the digestive and endocrine systems.

Come into ustrasana by kneeling on your mat. You may want to have padding under the knees if it is more comfortable. Have the knees hip width apart and thighs perpendicular to the floor (Figure 7.29). Place the palms of the hands at the small of the back, fingers pointing downward. Draw the elbows toward each other and roll the shoulders back (Figure 7.30). Lift the heart upward and press the shoulder blades into the back of the ribs. Begin to arch the spine (Figure 7.31). If you are comfortable, you can stay here, hips forward, back arched. If you want to go further, remove one hand at a time and place your hands on your heels. You may wish to tuck the toes to bring the heels closer to the hands. Continue arching the spine and straighten the arms. Allow the heart to continue to lift upward. You can keep the neck in a neutral position or drop the head back (Figure 7.32). Do what is comfortable for you. Do not strain the neck or throat. Breathe. Stay here for up to a minute. Come out of camel by bringing one hand at a time to the hips. Rest in child's pose afterward (Figure 7.70).

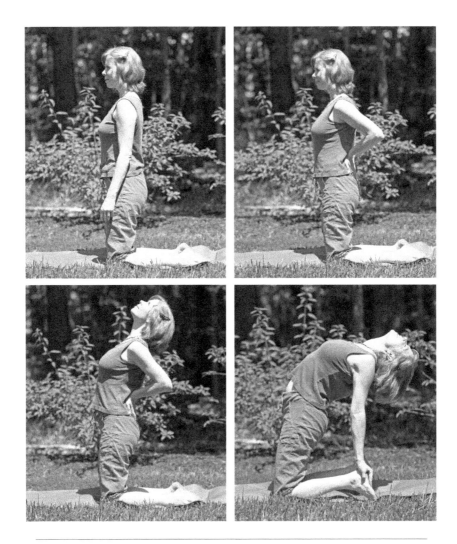

Figure 7.29 (1) Kneeling.

Figure 7.30 (2) Hands to small of back.

Figure 7.31 (3) Dropping the head, lifting chest.

Figure 7.32 (4) Full utrasana posture.

Bridge pose—Setu bandhasana

setu=dam or bridge *bandha*=lock

Bridge pose helps to strengthen the back, legs and hips. It opens the hips, the chest and the heart areas. It provides a calming and grounding energy and helps alleviate stress. It calms the brain and eases fatigue and anxiety, and stimulates the thyroid gland. Bridge pose can also help rejuvenate tired legs and a tired back. The pose lengthens the entire front of the body and helps to create space between vertebrae. Never practice bridge pose if you have neck injuries.

Lying on your back, bend the knees and bring the heels as close as possible to the buttocks (Figure 7.33). Hips, knees and ankles should be aligned. Place the palms of the hands on the floor alongside the hips. From here, press the lower back into the floor and tilt the tailbone toward the floor, noticing the motion of the pelvic tilt. You can do this motion several times to loosen the lower back. Pressing the lower back into the floor, roll the tailbone upward and continue to create an arch in the lower back vertebra by vertebra. Lift the hips as high as is comfortable, keeping knees, hips and ankles aligned. If you wish to move farther into the pose, walk the shoulder blades together, bringing the weight higher onto the shoulders. Bring the hands together under the arch of the body and interlace the fingers. Spread the chest and bring the chin toward the chest. If you wish, you can walk the feet closer to the buttocks to increase the arch (Figure 7.34).

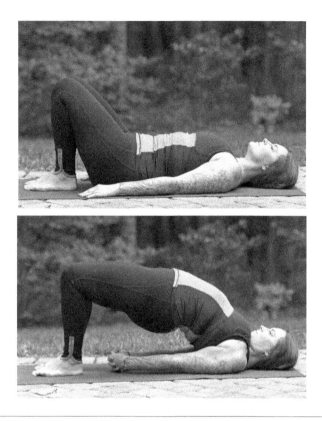

Figure 7.33 (1) Knees up, heels toward bottom.

Figure 7.34 (2) Bridge posture.

Supported bridge pose

Supported bridge posture, using a yoga block at the sacrum (Figure 7.35), "re-sets" the sacroiliac (SI) joint as well as the sympathetic nervous system, helping to facilitate a shift from stressed to calm.

For women who have experienced the death of a child at any age, due to any cause, during pregnancy or afterward, this supportive posture can help to create a sense of loving support around the sacral area. In my experience of practicing energy work with grieving mothers, the sacral chakra is very often the site of trauma, regardless of the child's age at death.

Overwhelmingly, grieving mothers have imbalances in the sacral chakra area and residual effects of trauma, emotional as well as sometimes physical.

Mothers hold energy from each pregnancy and birth in the sacral chakra, Svadisthana. When our children die, that energetic space is greatly impacted. Our womb space grieves this loss. This can manifest in physical pain and cramping in the uterine area, spontaneously crossing the arms over the abdomen in protective movements, and deep emotional pain centered in the sacral chakra space. These same kinds of physical and emotional pain, as well as energetic imbalances, can be held in the sacral space for survivors of sexual abuse and trauma. Supported bridge pose can create a sense of this chakra space being lovingly held, supported and in this support given the freedom to expand and open. As you inhale, imagine white or orange light spiraling around your sacral chakra. As you exhale, imagine stress, pain and anguish leaving this sacred space.

Hold supported bridge pose restfully for at least a minute, or longer if it's comfortable. Choose whatever height level feels most comfortable to you. You may also wish to lift the feet upward in this posture for a variation (Figure 7.36). To come out of the posture, place the feet onto the Earth, lift the hips, remove the block gently, and ease your lower back and hips back to the Earth. You may wish to practice yoni mudra (see Figure 4.2) for several breaths following this practice.

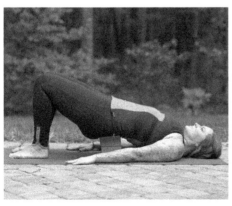 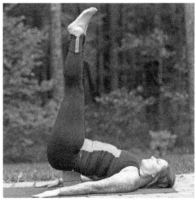

Figure 7.35 (1) Supported bridge with a block.

Figure 7.36 (2) Supported bridge, legs lifted.

Standing and balancing poses

These asana increase strength, balance and flexibility. They help us to feel strong, steady, balanced, energized and grounded. We can imagine untapped potential power residing in our legs, rooting us deeply into the Earth. Many of the names of these asana reflect the strength and groundedness we can experience in standing and balancing postures—the unity and balance of the triangle, strength of trees and mountains, grace and power of dancers and warriors, inspiration and intensity of the eagle. In standing poses, explore the postures as they find expression in you and allow their unique qualities to speak to you in body, mind and spirit.

Triangle pose—Trikonasana

tri=three *kona*=angle

Many yoga teachers say to imagine you are sandwiched between two panes of glass to keep correct alignment in this pose. How many of us feel that way in grief? Walled in, separated from the world by an invisible and impenetrable yet fragile barrier? This pose can help us transform that feeling of limitation to one of balance, strength and openness. The energy of trikonasana is that of reaching and extending. In this posture, what might you be reaching for? Help, support, hope, love, connection? In the extension, where and how might you need or want to extend yourself? Where might you be extending or pushing yourself too far? Reach or extend further than your own edge and you will be off balance.

In trikonasana we are challenged to maintain the equilibrium of our center of gravity—grounding through our feet, the base of the triangle, while reaching outward and upward, holding all three directions in balance. In trikonasana, where is your balance steady? Where is it not? The goal is not to have a perfect pose but to notice where you might be unsteady and adjust so that you are more balanced. Notice what you might need to do to bring more stability and comfort to your posture. Where might you extend just a bit further and how much is too much? If the extension either outward or upward is too much, the balance and steadiness of the base of the posture will be thrown off. Do you need to extend a little less to stay comfortable? Do you need a block for support in maintaining balance?

Recognizing your own needs is part of adapting, adjusting and accommodating. This is true in life and in all yoga poses. In trikonasana, perhaps more than any other standing pose, we are challenged to notice these things—extension in opposition or harmony with balance. Trikonasana opens the hips and the chest, elongates the spine, tones the muscles of the legs and the intercostal muscles of the rib cage. In it we can feel expansion, groundedness and freedom of spirit.

To practice trikonasana, have the feet about three feet apart, find the stance that is comfortable for you. Turn the right foot outward about 90 degrees. Turn the left foot in about 45 degrees. Be sure that you can move your hips freely. If you cannot, adjust your stance. The legs should form a triangle with the floor as the base. Inhaling, raise the arms to shoulder height and move the shoulders away from the ears (Figure 7.37). Shift the hips to the left, as if you have a string attached to that hip and it is being pulled away from you, and at the same time reach outward with the right arm. Imagine the left hip and right arm being pulled in opposite directions as far as is comfortable for you (Figure 7.38). Maintaining alignment, lower your right hand toward your right shin, moving toward the ankle. Place your hand on a block, adjusting the height as needed. Bring the left hand overhead, palm facing forward. Rotate the top shoulder back. Keep the hip bones facing forward. Remember the image of keeping the body sandwiched between two panes of glass. If it is comfortable, gaze up to the lifted arm. If this strains the neck in any way, gaze forward or down. To come out of trikonasana, raise the torso, lower the arms and bring the feet together. Repeat trikonasana on the other side.

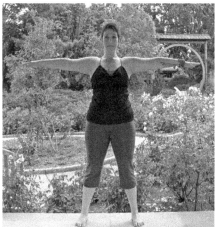
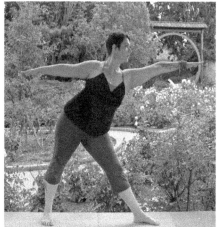
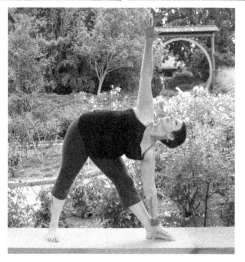

Figure 7.37 (1) Wide leg/arms out.

Figure 7.38 (2) Hip back, arm forward.

Figure 7.39 (3) Trikonasana.

Warrior I, II and III—Virabhadrasana I, II, III

virabhadra=mythical warrior created by Shiva

Easily one of the most iconic and recognizable postures, warrior pose serves to remind us of our own power. The pose is named for the mythological warrior Virabhadra, whose name means "blessed hero." Virabhadra was created by the God Shiva when he found the lifeless body of his love Shakti. Shakti had been deeply hurt and rejected by her father Daksha. Upon her father's failure to recognize her as the Supreme Goddess, Shakti left the world rather than live in a place where she was spurned. Shiva was nearly mad with grief. He tore his hair and threw the great black locks to the Earth, where they exploded with thunder and fire. The great warrior Virabhadra rose from the flames of Shiva's grief and rage. Virabhadra raised a great army against Daksha. Many were killed. Daksha's head was severed. His wife was left widowed and their other children fatherless. Eventually, Shakti returned to her body and all was restored, as things are in the worlds of gods. The story of Virabhadra's fierceness serves to remind us of the immense power of grief, and the destruction that can be wrought when such powerful energy is loosed. The posture embodies the energy of the spiritual warrior, the archetype evident in the story of Virabhadra who did battle with not just Daksha, but with ignorance and the power of mindless ego, the roots of Daksha's thoughtless disdain toward his daughter, the embodiment of the Goddess.

Warrior pose brings the opportunity to feel and observe your warrior energy. It asks you to experience your own power, which can rise from the challenges of life. In the posture, sink into that power. Contemplate what it might mean to turn the strength of your grief from destruction to creation, from chaos to balance. Emotionally, this posture helps to facilitate courage and bravery. It is excellent for days when we are fearful that we cannot do this—whatever *this* may be. We can use the strength of both Shiva and his warrior Virabhadra to help us draw upon the fire of our grief and our struggles throughout life and find a way to begin to draw strength from the transformative nature of the very things which have caused so much pain. This pose balances Muladhara, the root chakra, and helps us to feel more secure and grounded in our own strength and power.

To move into Warrior I from tadasana, exhale and step the feet to about four feet apart, finding a distance that feels comfortable for you. If you are on a yoga mat, the outer edges of the feet should be parallel to the short ends of your mat. Raise the arms upward overhead, bringing the biceps alongside the ears. If this strains the neck or shoulders, bend the elbows. Turn the left foot inward to the right, about 45 degrees. Turn the right foot outward 90 degrees, pointing toward the end of the mat. Rotate the torso toward the right toes, squaring the hips toward the toes. Adjust your foot position, rotating the left foot further inward if needed for stability and comfort. Recall the motion of cat/cow, and the pelvic rock in bridge pose, and engage that same motion, lengthening the tailbone toward the floor. Arch the upper back slightly. Grounding the left heel firmly, exhale and bend the right knee. Check to be sure the knee is not extending outward over the toes. You may also adjust your footing or stance here. You will work toward having the right thigh parallel to the floor. If it feels comfortable, reach strongly upward, spread the palms wide, facing each other, or bring the hands together. Arch back slightly and gaze upward if this is comfortable (Figure 7.40). Hold the posture for 30 seconds to 1 minute, contemplating your strength within with each breath.

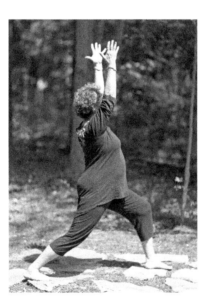

Figure 7.40 Warrior I.

From Warrior I, you may return to tadasana, or move directly into Warrior II. To move into Warrior II, rotate the torso from the front-pointing toes, to center, opening the arms as you turn, so that they become parallel to the floor. The foot stance is essentially the same, but adjusted slightly so, rather than being grounded in the left heel, the grounding is along the outer edge of the left foot. Ensure that the hip points now face center, aligned with the long edge of the mat. Center the torso. Check that you are not leaning toward the bent right knee. Have the right shin perpendicular to the floor, knee above the ankle. Imagine that someone is pulling your left arm gently, moving the torso to the center. Turn the head toward the right and gaze gently out across the right middle finger, finding your drishti point, a fixed spot, in the distance. Release the shoulders away from the ears (Figure 7.41). With each exhalation, sink a little deeper into the strength of the posture, finding a sense of relaxation within the intensity. From Warrior II, return to tadasana to rest. To prepare for Warrior III, move back into Warrior I. You can also move into Warrior III from a high lunge posture.

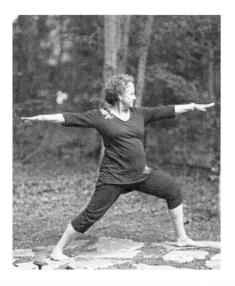

Figure 7.41 Warrior II.

To move into Warrior III, return to Warrior I. From Warrior I, fold the torso toward the bent leg, coming into a high lunge posture (see Figure 7.5). From your lunge, bring the arms forward so that they are parallel to each other, palms spread and facing each other. Simultaneously, straighten the front leg while lifting the back leg. The arms, torso and the raised leg should be as parallel to the floor as possible. Place the fingertips on the floor or on blocks for balance, raising them when ready. Hips point downward toward the floor (Figure 7.42). If there is shoulder or neck tension, feel free to adjust the arms, opening them outward if needed.

To come out of the pose, release the raised leg back to a lunge. Inhaling, step or walk forward into uttanasana, forward fold. Rest here for a few breaths and then, inhaling, bend the knees slightly, rise back up to tadasana. Repeat each posture, or the sequence of I, II, and/or III on the other side. You can also perform Warrior III with a chair for support (Figure 7.43). This can help with extension of the leg and working toward parallel positioning.

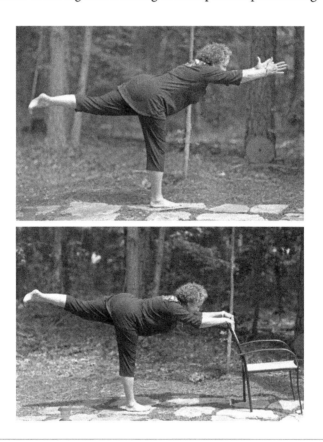

Figure 7.42 Warrior III.

Figure 7.43 Warrior III with chair for support.

Tree pose—vrksasana

vrksa=tree

Strong, beautiful, flexible, grounded, soaring—what kind of tree are you? This pose helps to create a feeling of balance and harmony on all levels. Tree pose helps us to feel grounded and supports the root chakra, Muladhara. In tree pose, you may wish to imagine roots growing from your feet into the ground, pushing into the floor, through the foundation of the building, into to soil of the Earth, past all the layers of rock, deeper and deeper into the Earth's crust until it reaches the red molten core of the planet. Imagine with each inhalation drawing this red light upward into your roots into the root chakra bringing strength, stability, warmth and security. As you exhale, allow fear, tension and stress to leave the body.

To come into tree pose, come first to tadasana. Find your balance and stillness first here. You may leave the arms down, have them on the hips, or together at the heart center in anjali mudra. Bring your awareness to the right leg and transfer the weight onto that foot, feeling the shift. Balance evenly, spreading the foot, distributing the weight evenly. Bend the left knee, externally rotating the hip so the knee points outward. Lift the left leg off the floor, placing the foot on the inside of the standing right leg (Figure 7.44). Place the sole of the foot on the ankle, the calf or the inner thigh of the right leg. Do not place the foot on the knee joint. To place the foot on the inner thigh, use the hands to position the foot properly. This can be a further challenge to maintaining balance. Once the leg is in place, bring the hands to anjali mudra. Keep the hands here, open into padma mudra (see Figure 3.7), extend the arms overhead clasping the hands, index fingers pointing upward in *vajra* mudra (Figure 7.46), or spread the arms wide like branches of a tree (Figure 7.45). Have the palms open in a receptive gesture. This posture is also a lovely pose in which to experience gratitude for the blessings of the Universe. Repeat the tree posture on the other side.

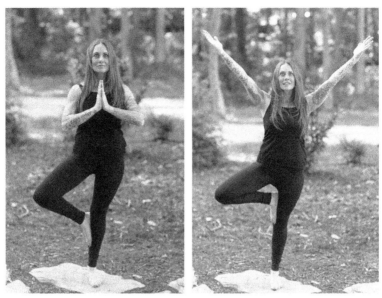

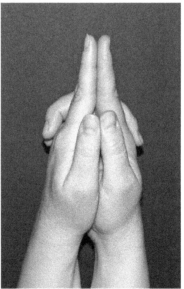

Figure 7.44 (1) Tree pose with anjali mudra.

Figure 7.45 (2) Tree pose, arms open.

Figure 7.46 (3) Vajra mudra, also known as "thunderbolt,"
opens sushumna nadi and moves energy upward.

King dancer—Natarajasana, also called Lord of the Dance pose

nata=dancer *Raja*=king

Nataraja is another name for the Hindu God Shiva, whose energy we also meet in Virabhradasana. In the trinity of major Hindu Gods, Brahma is Creator, Vishnu the Preserver, and Shiva the Destroyer. Shiva's universal dance of destruction is one of annihilation of the old, paving the way for newness and change. Without Shiva, there can be no creation of anything new. In many stories, Shiva's assistance is sought by the other gods who need his power to remove those things which no longer serve the ongoing growth, change and unfolding of the universe. He has many forms and, in his form of Nataraja, his dance represents the continual unfolding of life, death and rebirth. In this form he is represented as crushing the demons of ignorance, illusion and forgetfulness beneath his strong standing foot. Within the power of Shiva's pose, we can find the strength and grace to move with life's changes as well as facilitate the ability to create change in ourselves. Balanced on one foot, we can imagine crushing our own demons of ignorance, lack of awareness and lack of knowledge of our own strength and purpose. This posture is wonderful for increasing our balance and equilibrium as well. It opens the hip flexors and the chest, and stretches the abdominal muscles as well as the quadriceps.

To come into Natarajasana, begin in tadasana. Choose a drishti point, an immobile spot on the floor or the wall. This will help keep your balance and the mind steady. Shift your weight to the left foot. Find your balance on one foot. Lift the right foot and take hold of the right foot or ankle in your right hand. Stay here for a moment until you feel steady. Lift the chest and relax the shoulders. Raise the left arm toward the ceiling. You may stay here if you wish. To extend the pose, push the right foot/ankle into the right hand. To move deeper into the pose, simultaneously lengthen the torso and upward stretching arm, while lifting the right leg back and up, pressing the foot/ankle into the hand. As the torso shifts, keep the center of gravity above the standing leg to avoid tipping forward. Continue to feel the energy grounding downward through the standing leg, keeping the thigh firm, while lifting and reaching with the torso, extended arm and leg (Figure 7.47). To come out of the pose, perform the same movements in the opposite order, slowly, internalizing the balancing and focusing energy of this pose. Repeat the posture on the other side.

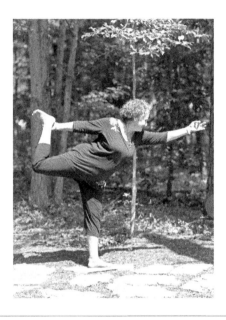

Figure 7.47 Natarajasana.

Eagle—Garudasana

Garuda=a fierce bird of prey, also the vehicle of the
Hindu god Vishnu, the Preserver of the Universe

This pose facilitates the energy of the eagle within. The spirit of Eagle posture allows us, in our mind's eye, to serenely soar above, focused, far-seeing, balanced. "Eagle-eyed" means able to see clearly, to have a keen ability to observe or watch, as well as to be able to see from far distances. The mythical humanoid birds known as the Garuda had magical abilities to fly without ever tiring. They could fly and ride the shifting changes of the winds endlessly if they wished. This pose can give us the ability to increase our insight and to cultivate the ability to ride the winds of change. Garuda is also the *vahana*, or vehicle, of Lord Vishnu the preserver and protector of all creation and the Hindu god of peace.

This pose also relates closely to the energy of the sixth chakra, Ajna chakra, the third eye, or brow chakra. Just as the vision of the mythic bird is limitless and timeless, our intuitive sight can also operate this way. In yoga, the third eye chakra is also associated with manas, the mind. Focusing on the balancing posture of Garudasana, you may notice that you cannot see anything at all beyond your entwined arms which block your physical line of sight. The posture asks that we move beyond typical vision into a space where our mind's eye can roam, seeing far. From Garudasana, we can sink into the groundedness of the posture while soaring in our mind's eye, seeing beyond obstructions, moving past even the mind and further into a space of wisdom and intuition. In addition to all the benefits of other standing and balancing poses, Garudasana opens the upper back and the shoulders as well as strengthens the thighs and ankles.

From tadasana find your balance and bring the hands either to the hips or to anjali mudra. Shift the weight to the right foot and bend the legs slightly. Lift the left foot and cross the left knee over the right. With the left toes toward the floor, press the left foot back and wrap the left foot behind the right calf. If the foot will not wrap around the calf, this is okay. Bend a little deeper and allow the toes of the left foot to touch the floor beside the outer edge of the right foot. Eventually, the foot will wrap around.

Stretch the arms forward until they are parallel to the floor and cross them at the elbows, right elbow above the left. Bring the hands upward and entwine the arms so that the palms face each other. If the palms do not come together, bring the fingers of the right hand into the palm of the left. Lift the elbows and stretch the fingers toward the ceiling (Figure 7.48). Hold the pose for 15 to 30 seconds. Breathe. To come out of the pose, unwind the arms, uncross the legs, return to tadasana, center the body and repeat on the other side.

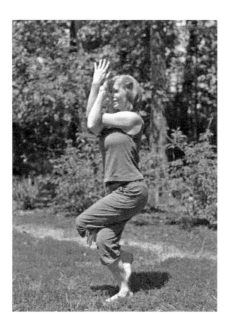

Figure 7.48 Garudasana.

Spinal twists

Spinal twists help increase spinal flexibility, relieve tension in the back and neck, and help regulate digestion. As the twisting action physically helps the body to release toxins through increasing lymph flow and massaging organs, we can imagine "wringing" out emotions we may prefer to be relieved of—anger, frustration, fear or simply stress in general.

Emotionally and spiritually, twisting to the left allows us to acknowledge our past. Twisting to the right encourages us to look toward the future. Coming back to center after twisting toward each side symbolizes recognition that we are living in the present moment, honoring what is here and now.

Revolved chair—Parivrtta utkatasana

parivrtta=to turn around *utkata*=fierce

This posture asks us to engage with two asana, utkatasana and revolved utkatasana. Utkatasana, so often referred to as "chair pose," translates as "fierce pose" but is often also called "awkward pose." Thinking of it as "awkward pose" can be a good metaphor for how we feel as we move through life in grief. Uncomfortable, self-conscious, uneasy, graceless, all good synonyms for awkward and for ways we can feel in grief. Learning to be comfortable in discomfort is also a great metaphor for the strength we can develop both physically in the awkward chair posture as well as in grief and other trials of life. As we sit in the awkwardness, we can cultivate strength and endurance.

Physically, this posture uses and builds strength in the ankles, the calves, the thighs, the back and the core, all of which lead to greater balance, better ability to move from our center, increasing feelings of groundedness and safety as we move through the world. In the posture and in grief, even as we develop tolerance and strength, we can continue to feel incredibly awkward and uncomfortable. The deeper the seat of the chair (the squat), the more the body must resist gravity. As we move through the world in grief, we often find ourselves struggling to resist the pull and the force of that pain. Chair and revolved chair poses can help us physically, energetically and emotionally strengthen our reserves and all the koshas to persevere when we find ourselves out of balance and torporous, being pulled downward toward the Earth, physically, energetically and metaphorically. This is a natural feeling in grief, but one that we can grow tired of. This pose can greatly help counteract those qualities of grief.

To move into utkatasana, come to tadasana. You may have the feet together or as much as hip width apart, whatever is more comfortable for you. Bring the arms overhead, perpendicular to the floor. If this creates stress for the neck or shoulders, open the arms by bending them at the elbows. Bend deeply at the knees, exactly as if you were about to sit down on a chair, knees pointing forward. The knees will extend out past the toes. Tuck the tailbone slightly, as if doing a micro cat movement in cat/cow pose (Figure 7.18), but maintain a small arch in the lower back. Keep the legs parallel to one another (Figure 7.49). To come out of chair pose, lower the arms, straighten the legs and return to tadasana.

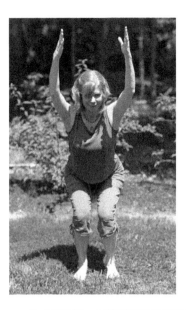

Figure 7.49 Chair pose—utkatasana.

Twisting in utkatasana adds the benefit of a twisting posture and brings a soothing quality to the pose and a unique sense of lightness. To twist and revolve in utkatasana, bring the hands from overhead into anjali mudra (Figure 7.50). This brings the awareness to the heart center and calms the brain. As you twist in prayer position, allow the movement in the posture to call up a sense of gratitude (Figure 7.51). Finding gratitude in our life while in deep grief can be a challenge, but can also be incredibly freeing. If you wish, open the arms wide in the twist to cultivate a sense of lightness and receptive quality to the posture. Emotionally, this asana helps to create a sense of peace and paradoxically, both stimulates and calms the nervous system, bringing a sense of invigoration as well as relaxation.

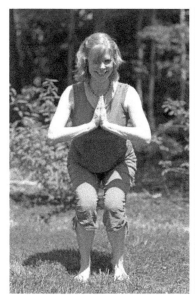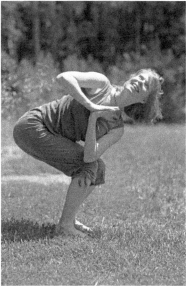

Figure 7.50 (1) Utkatasana with anjali mudra.

Figure 7.51 (2) Parivrtta utkatasana.

Half seated spinal twist—Ardha Matsyendrasana
ardha=half *matsya*=fish *indra*=ruler or lord

This posture is based on a Hindu story of Matsya, a fish who happened to be swimming by in the primordial ocean when Lord Shiva was explaining the Union of Yoga to the Goddess Pavarti. Matsya was enthralled and became very still, arching his spine upward to float as close to the surface as possible so he would not miss a word of the teaching. As he became more enthralled, he was effortlessly floating above the water. As he lost his fish consciousness, he became one with the consciousness of Shiva and of all existence. When Shiva recognized this, he touched Matsya and gave him a blessing that turned Matsya instantly human. He was then called Matsyenda, Lord of the Fishes. As he sat near Shiva and Pavarti to continue to hear the teachings, he sat in a way that helped to keep his mind and body calm. It is said that posture is the twisting pose of ardha matsyendrasana.

This pose gives a vigorous twist to the entire spine, tones and calms the nervous system and relieves pain and stiffness in the hips. To come into the posture, begin seated on the floor in dandasana, staff pose (Figure 7.52). Extend both legs out, spine lengthened. Roll the shoulders up, back and down, arms at the sides. Walk the buttocks back a bit to ensure that you're sitting squarely on your sitting bones. If your back rounds or your hips are uncomfortable, sit on a folded blanket.

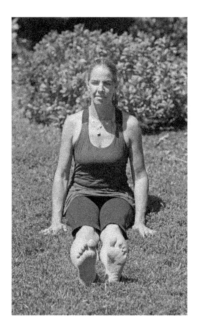

Figure 7.52 Dandasana.

Cross the right foot over the left and place the right foot on the outside of the extended leg where ever is comfortable for you. Some people think that they must have the leg that is crossed over very high up the thigh of the extended leg, but this is not the case. The goal is to be able to twist deeply. Some people may be able to twist more deeply with the crossed leg further down the outside of the extended leg. You may keep the leg extended (Figure 7.54) or bend it tucking the heel of the left foot near the right hip (Figure 7.53). Do whichever is most comfortable for you.

Once the foot of the bent knee is placed, take hold of the upraised knee with both hands and hug it in toward the body, stretching the spine upward. Twisting to the right, place the right hand behind you as close to the buttocks as possible, fingers pointing away from the body. Hug the knee, or place the left arm between the chest and upraised knee to use the arm as leverage. Twist the spine to the right. Initiate the twist first from the lower back, then middle, then upper and then the neck and head. Look over the right shoulder as far as is comfortable. Where the eyes go, the body follows. Imagine the spine as a spiral staircase twisting upward.

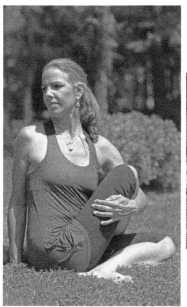 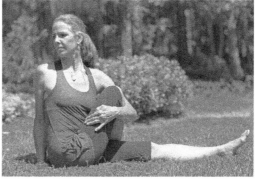

Figure 7.53 (1) Ardha matsyendrasana.

Figure 7.54 (2) Ardha matsyendrasana with leg extended.

With each inhalation, find a little more length in the spine, and with each exhalation, twist just a bit deeper, relaxing into the posture. To come out of the pose, untwist in the opposite direction, first the head and neck, upper, middle and then low back. Release the knee, stretch out both legs. You may want to do a minor counter twist in the opposite direction before setting up the pose to twist fully in the opposite direction.

Lying spinal twists—Supta matsyendrasana

matsyendrasana=Lord of the Fishes pose *supta*=reclining

Spinal twists done lying down can be very relaxing and calming and are a good way to end an asana practice as well as a nice wake up in the morning to get the spine moving and more flexible.

To practice, lie on the back. Draw the knees into the chest. You may wish to rock side to side here, giving the back a light massage. Extend the left leg downward while keeping the right knee bent. Extend the right arm outward at shoulder height, and holding the knee with the left hand, allow the right knee to fall toward the left side of the body. You can use the left hand and arm as leverage to help the right knee toward the floor. Turn the head to gaze to the right, keeping the right shoulder as close to the floor as possible (Figure 7.55). To come out, bring the knee back to the chest and then bring both knees into the chest. When you are ready, repeat the twist to the opposite side.

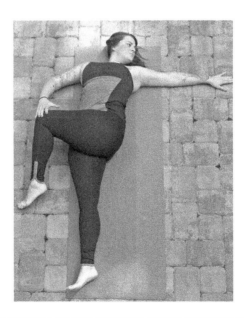

Figure 7.55 Lying spinal twist, leg extended.

Another version of the lying spinal twist is to practice the posture with both knees bent. Begin lying down and bring the knees into the chest. When you are ready, release both arms to the sides at shoulder height and with the knees bent, allow the knees to fall toward one side of the body. Gaze in the opposite direction. Again, keep the shoulders as close to the floor as possible. When you are ready, bring the knees back in to the chest, pause, and then allow the knees to fall to the opposite side (Figure 7.56). Release the twist when you are ready. Another variation is to cross the knees before allowing both knees to fall gently first in one direction and then the other. If you have the flexibility, you may try wrapping the foot around the opposite calf, coming to the leg position in Garudasana (Figure 7.48). Always gaze in the opposite direction to facilitate the twist.

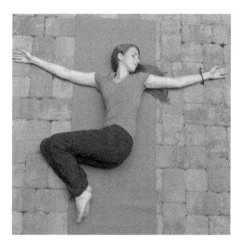

Figure 7.56 Lying spinal twist, knees bent.

Inversions and forward bends

All inversions calm the brain and promote a soothing feeling that is noticeable after coming out of the pose. An inversion is any yoga pose where the head is below the heart. They range from the fairly easy uttanasana, forward fold, to turning the entire body completely upside down in headstand or handstand.

Turning ourselves purposefully upside down may not sound like something anyone would want to do; when in grief, the world is already turned upside down. What would be the point in purposefully turning ourselves upside down in more ways? Turning ourselves in a completely different direction physically in a yoga pose can help us to imagine new metaphoric possibility and direction. Causing us to literally see the world differently, inversions can help us perceive the world, and ourselves, potentially and differently in ways other than what we are used to seeing.

Being upside down may not be for everyone. Anyone with unmedicated high blood pressure, certain heart conditions, recent stroke or eye problems such as glaucoma or detached retinas should not do inversions without discussing the risks with your doctor. Anyone with neck injuries should not do any inversion which puts pressure on the head or neck. In many yoga texts, women who are menstruating are advised against full inversions such as headstand, shoulder stands or handstands. Use caution and good sense.

Increased flow of blood to the brain increases concentration, induces calm and helps with mental functioning, including concentration, cognitive processing and memory. The lymphatic system can be greatly benefited by inverted postures and as a result the immune system can be supported. Inversions increase energy physically and mentally and help the circulatory system to function more efficiently. Inversions also increase balance and strength. They also help to improve confidence and overcome fear. They are also just plain fun. It's fun to be upside down! We can be playful and have fun in yoga and in life, despite being in grief.

Standing forward bend—Uttanasana

ut=intense *tan*=stretch

This pose encourages calmness and a deep awareness of the breath. From tadasana, place the hands on the hips, or if you wish, inhale the arms overhead. Allow the spine to lengthen. Fold forward from the hip joints, not from the waist. As you fold, lead with the heart to maintain length, keeping the neck a natural extension of the spine. If there is any stress in the lower back, bend slightly at the knees. As you fold, bring the abdomen toward the thighs. Allow the hands and arms to relax completely. Shake the head "yes" and "no" to release tension in the neck and allow the upper body to simply relax. Do not worry if the fingers or hands do not reach the floor. If you wish, place the hands on opposite elbows and allow the head to dangle in the space created there. On an exhalation, slightly contract the abdominal muscles to allow the back to release further. You may feel a slight spinal adjustment when you do this. If it is comfortable you may wish to wrap the arms around the calves, bringing the upper body closer to the legs. To create an energetic seal, you can come to *padahastasana*—hand under foot pose. In uttanasana, place the hands under the feet palms up, toes pointing toward the wrists.

See Figure 7.4 in the sun salutation series for uttanasa photo.

Downward facing dog—Adho mukha svanasana
adho=downward *mukha*=face *svana*=dog

Classic and widely recognized, the inverted "V" pose strengthens the arms and upper back as well as utilizing all major muscle groups. The energy of downward facing dog is active, but also receptive, counteracting anger and aggression. It is a posture of release and surrender, of rest and relaxation.

To practice downward facing dog, come to the hands and knees. You may wish to do a few rounds of cat/cow movement with the breath to loosen the spine and hips. From a neutral spine in table top position (Figure 7.16) have the hands and wrists slightly forward from the shoulders. The knees should be directly below the hips and calves parallel to each other. Spread the fingers and palms wide. Curl the toes under, exhale and lift the knees away from the floor and the hips upward. Keep the knees slightly bent. Come up to the toes and lift the sitting bones upward as if you were going to sit on the ceiling—again engaging the pelvic tilt experienced in cat pose. This brings the spine into the correct alignment. You may wish to pedal the heels one at a time, gently stretching the hamstrings, calves and ankles. When you are ready, bring the heels toward the floor. Only do what is comfortable for you. If you need to keep a bend in the knees or the heels slightly raised, do so.

Lengthen the spine and spread the shoulder blades. Allow the head to be relaxed, looking back toward the knees or your navel. Allow the breath to be rhythmic and easy. For a variation, try a three-legged dog, lifting the leg up and out, opening the hip flexors. From downward dog, you can practice coming into a lunge, and moving into pigeon pose.

To come out of adho mukha svanasana, return to the table top position. You may wish to take child's pose (Figure 7.70), or do a few cat/cow movements.

See Figure 7.6 for downward facing dog photo.

Handstand—Adho mukha vrksasana

adho=downward *mukha*=face *vrksa*=tree

Usually called "handstand," the Sanskrit actually means "downward facing" (adho mukha), or "upside down tree" (vrksa). This pose gives an entirely different perspective to everything. The whole self is literally turned upside down. Many people feel afraid to do this pose, even with the support of the wall, but feeling afraid and doing it anyway can help us to cultivate a sense of bravery in other aspects of our lives. Once you get the courage to try it, it can be incredibly rewarding. Handstands increase upper body strength, they are good for balance, especially freestanding handstands but, even when done against a wall, the posture requires full attention to what is happening in the body to remain properly balanced. It calms the brain and promotes a sense of feeling both restful and energized at the same time. Handstands also stimulate the pituitary and hypothalamus glands and help balance both Ajna, the third eye, and Sahasrara, the crown chakra.

You can come into handstand using a wall for support two different ways: facing toward or away from the wall. To begin facing away from the wall—which will end in an inversion with your face toward the wall—stand with your back against the wall. Bend forward and take downward facing dog with the backs of the heels to the wall. You may need to adjust your stance and your hands until you are in downward facing dog with the heels against the wall. Once you are here, begin to walk the feet up the wall. Initially, you will be in a wall-supported plank position. This position itself is a powerful inversion and brings the same benefits as a handstand. As you work to create a true vertical downward facing tree, you can adjust your placement and the walk as you feel comfortable eventually getting to a place where you can perform an inverted L-shape with the feet on the wall and the upper body vertically aligned. It can be helpful to have a partner watch and spot your alignment of wrists, shoulders and hips. Once you learn the feel of the wall-supported L-shape (Figure 7.57), you can begin to gently kick one leg off the wall at a time, coming into a vertical position.

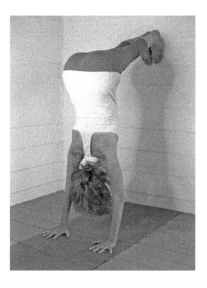

Figure 7.57 Inverted L-shape with wall support.

To come to handstand facing the wall—meaning you will be facing away from the wall once you come into the pose—face the wall and come to downward facing dog with the fingertips pointing toward the wall, about 12 inches away from the wall. Walking the feet closer in to the hands, shorten the stance of downward facing dog by about two thirds. This helps the upper body to be properly positioned when you kick up. Kicking your dominant leg up toward the wall, think of getting the hips over the shoulders rather than just the legs into the air. The non-dominant leg comes after, but also requires control. Negotiating space here can be challenging. It can be hard to understand where our bodies are in space when we are upside down. You may not know how far or close you are to the wall or to the floor. This is the proprioceptive sense and like all the senses, it can be challenged in grief. Handstand can help you regain a sense of your body and where it is in space.

You may need to practice gently kicking up and coming back down several times before you reach the wall. You may find that you're kicking too hard and bouncing off. Once your heels are up and against the wall, you can stay there and simply enjoy being upside down. When you feel comfortable, you can begin to bring the legs one at time away from the wall. Eventually you will be able to bring both away into the full handstand (Figure 7.58). Be prepared to fall. If you fall, try to maintain control with the arms so you don't crash. You may want to have a partner to help spot you and check alignment. Once you feel comfortable and strong enough, you might choose to attempt handstand with no walls. Do this from the shortened downward dog. Know that if you never do a handstand away from the wall, you still get the benefit from the full inversion. To come out of the posture, gently lower one leg at a time back to downward facing dog. Come to table top and either take child's pose (Figure 7.70) or come to standing. Hold handstand for a few seconds up to one minute.

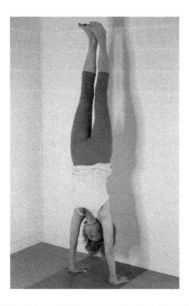

Figure 7.58 Handstand with wall from downward facing dog, fingers toward wall.

Shoulder stand—Sarvangasana or salamba sarvangasana

sarva=all *anga*=limb *salamba*=with support

Known as the Queen of Asana, shoulder stand brings many benefits. A sense of lightness and ease seems to suffuse the body. It is helpful for tired or swollen feet and legs. The posture helps with flexibility of the spine, strengthens the lower back and tones the abdominal muscles. It is known for its benefit to the thyroid, as the pressure on the gland causes thyroxine to be released into the bloodstream. Sarvangasana is very helpful before bed and helps to relax the entire body and the calm the mind. Shoulder stand is known to help balance and stimulate Vishuddha, the throat chakra. In this way, it can help us find our voices, speak our truth, express ourselves more clearly and also to be better able to listen and interpret the messages of others.

Sarvangasana is not recommended for those with uncontrolled high blood pressure, any neck or shoulder injury, glaucoma or recent surgery. The throat will be compressed during the posture. Do not talk or cough while the throat is compressed. If you are pregnant and have practiced shoulder stand before, it is fine to practice as long as you feel comfortable. If you've never practiced, it's not recommended that you begin while pregnant.

To come into sarvangasana, lie on the back. Bring the feet together and place the palms on the floor alongside the body. Pressing into the palms, bring the legs upward and overhead until they are parallel to the floor. Bring the palms of the hands to the small of the back to support the posture. You can bring the torso more perpendicular to the floor by walking the hands closer to the shoulder blades. Think of bringing the chest toward the chin. Bring awareness to the base of the throat. Breathe. Try to relax the neck and shoulders. If the cervical spine is uncomfortable, try shoulder stand with a folded blanket beneath the shoulders in supported shoulder stand (Figure 7.59).

To come out of shoulder stand, hinge from the hip joints and bring the legs overhead again until they are parallel to the floor. From here, you can practice *halasana*, plow posture, bringing the toes to the floor behind the head. Many people enjoy practicing plow pose after shoulder stand. To release the posture, bring the hands alongside the body, press the palms into the floor and, using the abdominal muscles, lower the legs gently.

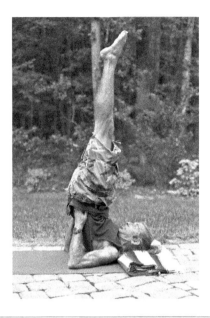

Figure 7.59 Sarvangasana, shoulder stand.

Forward bends

Forward bending postures bring our focus inward, promoting introspection and inner quietude. They help to draw the senses inward and can provide relief from the noise of the outside world. They can also help us to cultivate patience with ourselves, others and the world around us and they symbolize surrender and release. Just as the outwardly focused vulnerable energy of the backbending postures can give rise to difficult emotions, forward bends are more protective, but can give rise to awareness of inner turmoil. At times, it can be difficult to tolerate the thoughts and feelings that may be moving through us when we are in an inwardly focused posture.

Approached with awareness, seated forward bends help us to get better at letting go and surrendering into the experience of what is. Much emotional clearing can occur in seated forward bending postures. Done toward the end of a practice, they can help release tension and clear away emotional and energetic muck that may have been stirred up by other more active postures such as backbends and standing poses. Prana in seated forward bends moves inward and helps us to begin to draw our awareness inward as well.

The seated forward bends can often engage the pain of our inner child. These issues stem from deep seated and unconscious fears held at the base of the spine in Muladhara, the root chakra, as well pain from past relationships and unmet needs held in Svadisthana, the sacral chakra. Our fears of the unknown, fear of more loss, fear of death, fear of lack of connection with those we love—living and dead—can be stirred in these postures. The solar plexus chakra, Manipura, our place of personal power may also be affected. Physical, energetic, or emotional tension and resistance from the solar plexus and the sacral area all the way to the soles of the feet may rise. We may feel frustration, anger, deep sadness, fear or anxiety. With all yogic experiences try to remain aware and conscious of the experience, continuing to cultivate a witness consciousness with compassion.

Physically, forward bends create length and relieve compression in the spine, help us to be aware of the breath and bring our focus inward. Seated forward bends elongate the spine and also help to release and relieve stress and tension in the hips and hamstring areas.

Wide-legged standing forward bend— Prasarita padottanasana

prasarita=spread or expanded *pada*=foot *ut*=intense *tan*=stretch

This posture helps cultivate a sattvic state of balance. The lower part of the body is rooted, like a tree, legs strong and active, the upper body floating, spacious and tranquil, the pose embodies the harmony of energy and relaxation. This pose is also an inversion and very calming to the brain and the nervous system. Wide-legged standing forward bend helps balance Ajna, the third eye chakra and Sahasrara, the crown chakra. Because of the opening and balancing of those two upper chakras, this posture may hold far less of the fear, anxiety and sadness sometimes experienced in seated forward bends. Have yoga blocks available for resting the hands, elbows, or the head if you choose.

To move into this posture, begin in tadasana and step or hop the legs between three to four feet wide. Taller people will feel more comfortable with a wider stance. Find the position that is most comfortable for you. Press the outer edges of the feet and the big toes into the floor. Firm the thighs. Place the hands on the hips if this is comfortable for you. Inhale and extend and lengthen the spine, exhale and begin to fold forward. When the torso is parallel to the floor, place the fingertips or palms on the floor. Pause here to notice how you are feeling and continue to lengthen the spine. On an exhalation, continue to fold forward, leading with the heart. Come into a full forward fold that is appropriate for your body. Keep the shoulder blades wide and the shoulders moving away from the ears. You may choose to rest the crown of the head or your hands on a block. Some people may be able to rest the crown of the head on the floor (Figure 7.60). Every one of us is in a different body. Do what feels comfortable in your body. Stay here for 30 seconds to 1 minute.

To come out of the pose, bring the hands under the shoulders, lengthen and lift the torso. Once the torso is parallel to the floor, firm the thighs and root the feet, bring the hands to the hips and bring the torso all the way up. Lengthen the tailbone toward the floor and walk or hop the feet together. Stand in tadasana and notice how you feel.

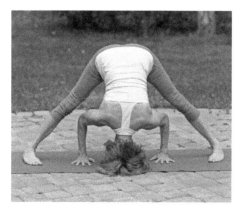

Figure 7.60 Prasarita padottanasana.

Head to knee pose—*Janu sirsasana*

janu=knee *shiras*=to touch with the head

Janu sirsasana asks that you bring the head toward one knee at a time, creating a slight asymmetry in the body's alignment and a subtle spinal twisting movement to the forward bending posture.

The pose can be emotionally difficult for some. Anger, fear or sadness may arise. Because janu sirsasana includes deep forward bending as well as twisting, deep emotional or energetic release can be increased. Continuing to lengthen the spine with each inhalation and relaxing further into the posture with each exhalation can help facilitate the release of any held energies. Think of the energy and emotion moving down and out of the koshas, being dispersed into the Universe, transformed into neutral energy.

To come into janu sirsasana, bring the legs together stretched out in front of the body into dandasana, staff pose (Figure 7.61). Walk the buttocks backward slightly to come forward onto the sitting bones. If it is more comfortable, sit on a folded blanket. This can help the sitting bones to be in the correct position and greatly assist the fold from the hip joint. Keeping the right leg extended, bend the left knee, bringing the sole of the foot to the inside of the right thigh as high up as is comfortable. Ideally, the heel should be aligned with the center of the body. If you have the flexibility and it feels comfortable, allow the heel to press against the body. This helps stimulate energy in the root chakra.

Inhale and bring the arms up alongside the ears, lengthening the spine upward. Ensure that the hips are squared and facing forward (Figure 7.62). Move slowly, breath by breath into the posture. Exhale, and arching the lower back slightly, lead with the heart and fold forward extending the torso out over the extended leg. Stop, inhale and lengthen the spine from the pelvis, lifting the rib cage. The sternum should be centered over the extended leg. Exhale and continue to fold slowly forward. Lengthen with each inhale, fold further with each exhale. When you reach your maximum extension, relax the upper body and allow the head to move toward the knee. Relax the arms, torso, neck and head. Allow the hands to rest anywhere they are comfortable, on the shin, the ankle, holding the foot, or on the floor. If you hold the foot or leg, you can continue to lengthen the spine on an inhalation, using the leg for leverage, relaxing with an exhalation (Figure 7.63). Notice that if you contract the thigh muscle slightly, the hamstring can release a bit further. Continue to breathe. You can stay here for up to three minutes.

To come out of the pose, look forward, past the toes, reach the heart forward, lengthening the spine once more, and rise up while inhaling. Stretch out both legs, perhaps give the spine a small counter twist the opposite side, set up dandasana once more and repeat the posture with the other leg extended.

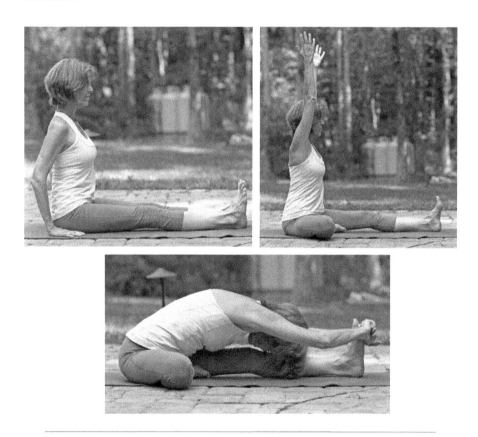

Figure 7.61 (1) Dandasana—staff pose.

Figure 7.62 (2) Lengthening spine, preparing to fold forward.

Figure 7.63 (3) Janu sirsasana.

Seated full forward bend—Paschimottanasana
pascha=behind, after, westward *uttana*=intense stretch

Paschimotanasana, "intense stretch of the west side of the body," is ideal to practice following janu sirsasana. The pose holds the same emotional qualities as all forward bends, moving the awareness inward, encouraging introspection and sense withdrawal. Be aware of rising emotions and sensations in this pose. Purposeful, conscious use of paschimottanasana can be helpful in releasing emotional pain from current relationships as well as from childhood, facilitating the release of energies from the root and sacral chakras. While in dandasana, preparing to move forward in the fold, imagine your inner child sitting on your own lap. Picture what you looked like as a child, innocent, open, trusting, seeking security, love and care. Think of all the things that your inner child may still be missing. As you sit, imagining your inner child on your lap, allow yourself to notice what feelings rise— fear, anxiety, longing, confusion. You don't have to know why the feelings are there, or even what may be attached to childhood, later relationships, or your current grief. Often current feelings invalidated by important people in our lives mirror those we experienced in childhood when we were not heard or validated. Sit for a moment with any feelings that may rise. If none do, still imagine your inner child there with you, still an integral part of who you are. Begin to send love from your heart space into the heart of your inner child. As you fold into the posture, visualize embracing and soothing that child, folding love inward while validating any emotions that rise from within. As you rest in the posture, allow the love to flow toward your inner child and any uncomfortable feelings to leave the body, heart and spirit with each exhalation.

From dandasana, inhale as you lengthen the spine, raising the arms overhead. As you fold forward, lead with the heart, looking forward, stretching outward over the legs. Slowly, as with janu sirsasana, exhale as you fold, inhale while reaching forward for a bit more length. When you reach your maximum extension, allow the hands to rest and the torso to rest (Figure 7.64).

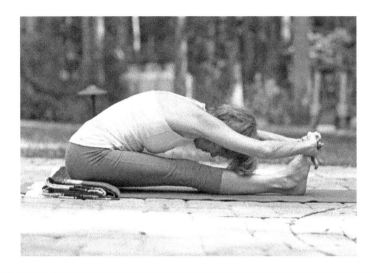

Figure 7.64 Paschimottanasana.

Hip opening postures

We may not immediately think of the hips as a space where deep emotional energy is stored, but this space is vital to emotional and creative health. For women, the hips are often the center of gravity, the very epicenter of who we are. For men, while the center of gravity is slightly higher, the hips and the pelvic area are the source of forward and directive movement. For both sexes, the hips and pelvic region are sites of trauma on many levels and from many sources, physical and energetic. The pelvis, groin, and hips are the center of creativity and sexuality for us all. Memories of childhood are stored in the cells of the large group of muscles known as the hip flexors, as well as energetically in Svadisthana, the sacral chakra. In this energetic center, all impressions of emotional relationships past and present are held.

We depend on our hips for survival and protection in more ways than we realize. From the instant of birth onward, our instinctive reflexes stimulate the body's flexors to draw the knees upward to shield the torso and the ribs inward to protect vital organs. This reflexive and protective movement can be seen in day-old infants. Our hips must be ready to help us kick, shield, run, dodge, dash, dart or stand firm whenever the fight, flight, freeze response is activated. Chronic stress results in prolonged tension in any muscle group, due either the repetitive physiological movement or psychological and emotional stress. Grief is a chronic state of stress. The instinctual reflexes of the hips are associated with protection and survival as well as potential trauma history. These things combined can result in tightness, pain, emotional instability and the inability to relax and release those muscles.

Experience of emotional releases in hip opening postures is very common. Know that if this occurs, it is not abnormal. Release occurs when the body feels safe. As with back and forward bending postures, see if you can remain present with whatever feelings arise, observing with compassion and love what is happening on all levels of your being.

Pigeon pose—Eka pada rajakapotasana
eka=one pada=foot raja=king kapota=dove or pigeon

This asana is ideal for practicing what Patanjali calls ishvara pranidhana, surrender to the Universe, to God, to circumstances, to whatever your body, as well as your heart, is feeling and capable of doing in this very moment in time. Physically, it is an excellent hip opener, helping to release stress and tightness in the hip area, where many of us carry a great deal of stress. Hip-related emotional catharsis is not unusual in this posture, or other hip opening postures.

Another aspect of pigeon posture is the association with the animal itself. Pigeons always know how to find their way home. Resting in this posture, surrendering to what is, we can allow our own homing instinct to rise, knowing that wherever we go, wherever we are, we are always home.

A good preparatory posture for pigeon pose is "thread the needle." Lying on the back, thighs parallel and hip distance apart cross the right ankle over the left thigh with the foot flexed to protect the knee. Bring the left knee toward the chest and reach the right hand through the space between the legs, the left hand around the outside of the left thigh and grasp either the back of the left thigh or the left knee with both hands. Choose the position that will allow the upper body to remain relaxed on the floor. Bring the left knee toward the chest while pressing the right knee away.

To come into pigeon, begin in downward facing dog or in table top posture. When you are ready, lift the right leg, bringing the knee between the hands. Place the knee slightly behind and toward the right wrist, the heel of the foot pointing toward the left hip. The shin of the right leg will face toward the front of the mat. The more parallel the right shin is to the front of your mat, the more intense the stretch to the hip. For less intensity, bring the heel toward the center of the body. Slide the left leg backward behind you, lengthening the leg as far as possible, allowing the quadriceps to release toward the floor. Ensure that both hip bones are facing forward. If you notice that your right hip is rolling downward, you can place a folded blanket or a block under the hip for support and to help the hips face forward. Use the arms for support as you set your body up for the posture rather than placing weight on the hips or twisting the lower back. The right leg is externally rotated and left is neutral (Figure 7.65). In this pose, you may feel intense stretch in the right hip, the right buttocks or the inner thigh. You should never feel discomfort in the knees. If there is any twinging, pressure or pain in the knee, come out of the posture. If there are no difficulties with the knee, lengthen the spine and begin to fold forward over the right shin.

Once you are in your maximum fold, try to relax into the posture (Figure 7.66). You may wish to support your head on a block or the upper body on a bolster or a stack of folded blankets. You may wish to take anjali or jnana mudra with the hands to help focus the mind. Remain in this posture for up to five minutes if you wish. If the sensations are intense, direct prana with each breath into the spaces of tenderness or rigidity, finding a place of stillness within.

To come out of the posture, bring the hands to the floor beneath the shoulders, inhaling, lengthen upward. Protecting the knee, roll gently onto the right hip and bring the left leg up to meet the right. You may wish to lie back and with both knees bent, feet on the floor, allow the knees to fall side to side, in windshield wiper motions. Set the pose up for the other side and repeat.

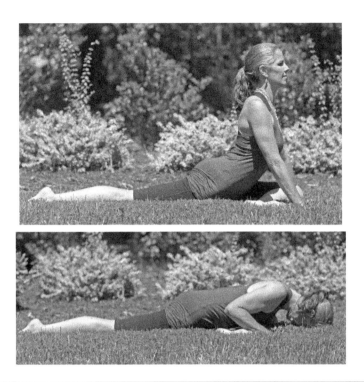

Figure 7.65 (1) Pigeon pose set up.

Figure 7.66 (2) Pigeon pose—Eka Pada Rajakapotasana.

Restorative poses

Restorative yoga is the practice of supported, passive postures. Once your body is in the posture, you simply rest there. Sensory stimulation is reduced; you may wish to dim the lights and practice in a quiet space, and use slow, calm, relaxing music that will not detract from the experience. If you can, use an eye pillow, a scarf or hand towel to cover the eyes and block out light, but only if this is comfortable. Most restorative postures will use supports like bolsters, blankets or pillows to help support the body, requiring no effort from the muscles. Typically you will remain in a restorative posture for at least five minutes or longer. Restorative postures can lower the heart rate and blood pressure, allow the body to rest, stretch the muscles and calm the nervous system.

Many people experience a restorative class or practice as near paradise, lying there doing nothing, allowing the pose itself to transport you to a place of relaxation and calm. Some can completely lose a sense of body awareness and enter into deep meditative states; for others, being still and purposefully restful can stimulate anxiety and stressful thoughts. In grief, you may find that, in a restorative pose, your mind goes back to memories of your loved one; increased feelings of loss and longing can arise. In a restorative posture, we are asking our bodies to release all tension and control of the muscles that we depend on when the nervous system shifts into the fight, flight, freeze mode. If you are experiencing anxiety and stressful thoughts, the body will respond. The experience can feel alarming or confusing. Often these kinds of feelings can be soothed by adding more props—blankets and bolsters— that help to increase a sense of groundedness and support. Ensuring that the limbs of the body feel supported in their sockets, that you are warm, that there is support beneath you, can counteract these kinds of experiences and promote a sense of comfort, of being held in a safe space.

Legs up the wall pose—Viparita karani

Viparita=contrary or reversed karani=doing or making

This posture is one of receiving and relief. It requires little effort and brings a great deal of comfort and calm. The posture has a very grounding, nurturing energy, increasing our ability to accept love, support and care. It helps with swollen feet and ankles, tired legs and back. It is particularly helpful for lower back pain and can help lymph drainage and circulation in the lower body. It is an excellent posture for helping with sleep and any time you feel a need to simply rest.

With your bottom as close to the edge of the wall/floor as possible, support yourself with your arms and bring your feet straight up the wall. Lie back onto the floor. This pose is very helpful before bed. It relieves swelling in the feet and legs and encourages relaxation. Emotionally, legs up the wall helps us to feel a liberated relief, that we may not have to work so hard all the time, that we can put our burdens down and accept that we are supported—

by others, by the Universe, by our own inner peaceful Selves. We can allow the flow of energy to be reversed.

Props (optional):

- 1–3 blankets

- bolster.

If you are using a mat, have the short end of the mat flush to the wall. If you are using blankets, fold the blankets four times and place them in a stack next to your mat. To come into the posture, sit sideways with knees bent and with the hips and buttocks as close to the wall as possible. Lie back and swing the legs upward, "walking" the body and bottom around until the buttocks are as close as you can get them to the wall. If this is too much stretch for the hamstrings, bend the knees a bit and scoot the buttocks slightly away from the wall. To add the support of the blankets, walk the feet down the wall and lift the hips. Place the blankets beneath the hips for support (Figure 7.67). For added groundedness, place a folded blanket across the hip bones. Notice what is happening in the mind and let the breath be easeful and slow. If your mind is racing, try to have the exhalation be longer than the inhalations.

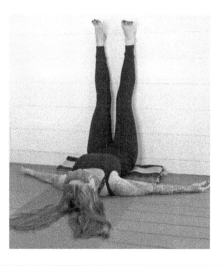

Figure 7.67 Viparita karani.

You may also wish to try this posture with the legs supported on a chair or low table (Figure 7.68). Ensure that the height of the chair or table is equal to or a little higher than your feet. Feel free to use a blanket for support under the hips as well as under the arms if you wish.

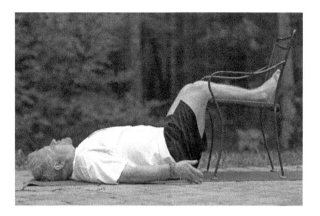

Figure 7.68 Legs on a chair.

Bound angle pose—Supta baddha konasana

supta=resting *baddha*=bound *kona*=angle

Props (optional):

- 1–3 blocks

- 1–5 blankets

- 1–2 bolsters

- 2–4 pillows

- 1 strap.

Supta baddha konasana, also known as supported butterfly, opens the throat, heart, chest, belly and pelvic spaces. These are the places that we protect the most. In this restorative posture, all of these are exposed and vulnerable. If you experience discomfort mentally or emotionally, try to slow the breathing, letting the exhalation be longer than the inhalation. Let the focus be on the breath. You may also choose to practice the *Come to Your Senses* exercise from the Pratyahara section of the Raja chapter.

To set up the posture, place a block lengthwise under a bolster to create an incline. Sit with your sacrum at the low end of the bolster. If you like, you can sit on one or two folded blankets for support under the hips and sitting bones. Lie back supported by the bolster and block. You can place a second bolster under your knees if you wish, or support the knees with pillows or yoga blocks. Place folded and stacked blankets or pillows under the elbows and forearms (Figure 7.69). The goal is to feel completely supported and held. To avoid having to work keep the soles of the feet together, you can secure the feet by wrapping a strap around the ankles. You may also place a folded blanket across the hip bones for a gentle, grounding pressure. Wrapping the feet with a blanket can also increase a sense of being held. You can choose to use all or only a few of these suggested props. Ensure that you feel supported and there are no active stretching sensations in the thighs, groin, chest or shoulder areas and no tension in the neck. Relax in this posture for up to 15 or 20 minutes.

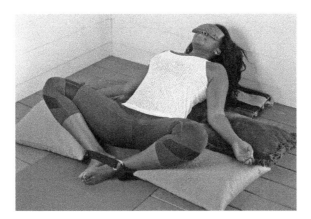

Figure 7.69 Supta baddha konasana.

Child's pose—Balasana

bala=child

In child's pose, you may feel your heart center swell. This swelling of energy and emotion may be noticeable at the front and the back of the heart, you may also feel it in your belly. If you can, simply allow the feelings to be what they are. If there are tears, allow this to be okay as well. In this pose, reach back in your history to when you were a child when you did not hold back emotions or tears, back to a time before you learned to hold them in and dry them up so as not to upset anyone else or to seem vulnerable or weak. In child's pose, allow whatever feelings arise to simply be what they are. If you feel safe, allow them to spill out onto the altar of your heart. Balasana is a pose of surrender and of rest. To surrender, to release, to give over the things that are too heavy to carry, too painful to hold in this moment, to lay them down, if even for a moment, can allow for deep rest.

This posture is essentially a fetal position. To practice child's pose, come to hands and knees and bringing the big toes together, sink the hips back toward the heels. Feel free to have the knees as wide as is comfortable for your body. Fold the upper body over the thighs and allow the arms to rest where ever is most comfortable for you, either overhead, forearms stacked or stretched out at your sides, toward the feet, palms up (Figure 7.70). This is a resting posture to which you can come at any time during asana practice or anytime you feel your inner child needs to be nourished and soothed.

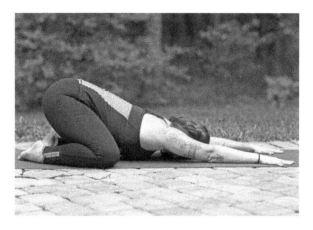

Figure 7.70 Balasana—Child's pose.

Corpse pose—Savasana

sava=corpse

Props: (optional)

- bolster

- hand towel.

Teachers say this is hardest pose of all. Allowing every muscle in our bodies to fully relax can seem a nearly impossible task. We must release emotionally and mentally in order to truly and completely relax physically. In this posture memory and emotion may also rise. This is a sign of release and safety. Emotional release will only occur if you feel safe enough to allow it. In savasana, the final pose of an asana class, the body is able to integrate the benefits and results of all the previous postures practiced.

In savasana, the body should be in a neutral position. To find the appropriate position for your body, bring the feet together and slowly move them apart to find the position with the least amount of tension. This is usually about shoulder width apart. Allow the feet to be splayed apart with no tension in the ankles or toes. Do the same with the arms and allow the palms to face upward. If the neck feels tense, use a rolled hand towel for gentle support under the neck. If the lower back is tense or if there is any discomfort there, place a bolster beneath the knees (Figure 7.71). If you do not have a bolster, bend the knees, bringing them together with the feet apart.

In savasana, from the toes to the head, mentally move through the body scanning for any areas of tension. If you find any areas of tension, send a mental message for those areas to totally relax. As you breathe, with each exhalation, send prana to the spaces where you feel any tension. Remain in savasana as long as you wish. Savasana is an excellent time to listen to guided meditations or to simply watch what is happening in your own mind, as always with compassion and without judgment. Allow the entire body to soften and notice where you may feel any sensations or movement of prana. You can also practice directing prana to various parts of the body, noticing what differences or changes you may experience.

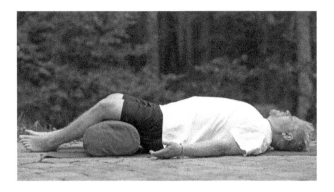

Figure 7.71 Savasana with bolster under knees for support.

Pranayama

Prana is the life force which moves everything in the Universe. Pranayama is the strengthening, cultivation, control and direction of prana. It is the vital force that connects, surrounds and suffuses everything. We receive the most amount of prana from and through our breath. Because our breath can be controlled, it is an ideal way to practice the control of prana in our own being. We begin with simple breathing practices and proceed to more advanced ones. The practices of pranayama are powerful. They can calm the body and soothe the mind, focus the attention and lift the spirits. The breath is the bridge between body and mind. Patanjali tells us in sutras 47–49 that with the practice of asana—comfortable and steady posture—comes a relaxation of effort which lessens the tendency for restlessness. From that, pranayama naturally follows. It works the opposite way as well, calm the breath, calm the body and calm the mind.

To begin, we must learn to become aware of the breath. Most of us are not breathing properly for optimum health and well-being. We have poor posture, we may sit at our desks or on sofas for long periods of time, craning our necks, staring at screens, generally moving very little. On top of that, grieving makes us feel like we want to be even further slumped, curled up and protecting our hearts. Our lungs are unable to expand fully and our breath, and prana, is even more restricted than normal.

Often when I ask someone to show me a deep breath, people automatically suck in their stomachs and fill up their chests; the opposite of a deep, full breath. That kind of breath restricts the lungs' ability to take in oxygen and release carbon dioxide. The result is an excess of CO_2 in the body. Too little oxygen and too much CO_2 can increase fatigue, mental fog and decreased tissue function. For a grieving person, this intensifies many of the normal grief reactions you are already dealing with. Breathing deeply and fully can decrease stress, increase clarity of thought, calm anxiety and help counteract fatigue.

Finding a quiet time at any point in your day to simply breathe can be a wonderful tool for self-care. Any time you notice that you are feeling anxious, particularly tired or that you are holding your breath, take a moment—right then and there—to breathe. Stop lights make good cues to practice your breathing as well. In addition to helping you notice your breath and serving as reminders to practice your breathing exercises, breathing at stop lights can help to counteract the stress we experience when we are confronted with the world. Noticing your breath and increasing your use of pranayama, with or without asana, can help you to become more mindful of your own thoughts and feelings, giving you a greater sense of control and stability in the chaos of grief.

Just breathe

This is an exercise in simply noticing your breath, becoming aware and mindful of your own breath as it moves in and out of your body. To begin, sit in any comfortable position, on the floor or on a chair, with your spine long and straight but not stiff. You can also practice this in savasana or any of the restorative postures. Find a comfortable position for your hands, either folded gently in your lap, or resting on your thighs or knees—palms up or down, whichever feels right to you. Close your eyes if that feels comfortable. If not, find a spot on the floor a few feet in front of you and allow your gaze to soften. As you sit, begin to notice the temperature of the air on your skin, notice any sounds you may hear within or outside the room. Begin to notice your body's weight as it is supported by the chair or the floor. Notice the feel of the floor or the chair under your sitting bones, under your legs. Notice the feel of the floor beneath your feet. Expand your awareness to noticing the sensations of your entire body without feeling the need to change anything. Simply notice.

Now, begin to notice and follow the movement of your breath as it moves in and out of your body, as you inhale and exhale. As you inhale, notice the temperature and the vibration of the air as it flows through your nasal passages, down your throat and trachea, on its way into your lungs. Notice the different sensations of your belly, your ribs, your chest as they expand. As you exhale, notice the temperature of the air, the movement of the tiny hairs of your nose, the feeling of your lungs empty of air as it leaves your body. Simply notice these things and any other sensations that occur as you continue to breathe, easily and naturally, in and out. Simply notice your breath as it moves in and out of your body without the need to change anything at all. Notice how your breath feels. Is it easy and effortless? Or labored and difficult? Does watching the breath seem natural or strange? Without judgment, and with as much compassion as possible, just breathe.

Simple deep breathing

As above, find a comfortable position with your hands relaxed, either in your lap or resting on your thighs or knees. Relax your shoulders. Pull them up toward your ears, roll them back and down, creating space between your shoulders and your ears. Allow your shoulders to relax.

Breathe normally in and out for a few breaths. Notice how your belly rises and falls easily as you breathe naturally. Your chest should not rise a great deal as you breathe in and out. If you like, place a hand on your abdomen to bring your attention to the movement.

When you are ready, breathe into the belly slowly. On the exhalation, breathe out slowly through your nose, counting to five. During this exhalation, tighten your abdominal muscles, and pull your diaphragm inward, toward your spine, squeezing all the excess air out of your body. When all the air is squeezed out, pause slightly, and inhale slowly again, to the count of five, allowing your belly to expand as you breathe in. If you are comfortable doing so, close your eyes and continue to repeat this easy deep breath, 5–10 times.

The three-part breath—Deergha swasam

The three-part breath is a specific breathing technique used in yoga practices. *Deergha swasam* means "complete breath." It can be very useful in times of stress or whenever you need to relax. This type of breathing stimulates the parasympathetic nervous system, the relaxation response, and allows your body and mind to more easily release stress and tension. Practicing the three-part breath before bed can be very helpful with sleep problems.

In typical breathing, we use only about one third of our lungs' capacity. With Deergha Swasam, we can increase the amount of oxygen we are taking in by up to 70 percent. This can be soothing to the mind and can induce almost immediate calm. If you feel dizzy or lightheaded while practicing the three-part breath, or any other breathing exercise, stop the practice immediately and allow your breathing to go back to normal. Find your comfortable sitting position, allowing your hands to be relaxed. The three-part breath may also be done lying down. To begin, inhale. Then, with your mouth closed, exhale slowly through your nose as you did with the simple deep breathing exercises, using your abdominal muscles to pull your diaphragm inward. Squeeze all the stale, excess air completely out of your lungs.

As you prepare for your next inhalation, imagine your upper body as a large pitcher. As you inhale, you are filling the pitcher from bottom to top. As you inhale, fill the diaphragm and lower belly, allowing them to expand and completely fill with air. Next, continue to allow the pitcher to fill as you notice the lower, and then the upper, parts of the ribcage expanding outward and up. Finally, fill the upper lungs, noticing the chest expanding, the collarbones and shoulders rising, as the pitcher is filled completely to the top. Pause for two counts.

Exhale in the opposite way, allowing the pitcher to empty from top to bottom. As you slowly exhale, allow the shoulders and collarbones to slowly drop, the chest to deflate and the ribs to move inward. Pull your diaphragm in, using it to completely empty the air from the bottom of the lungs. Repeat the process, refilling the pitcher slowly from bottom to top. Continue with complete and full exhalations and inhalations, emptying and filling your pitcher.

The three parts are bottom, middle, top—expanding as you slowly and completely fill your body with fresh, cell-nourishing, life-giving oxygen and then contracting slowly as you rid the lungs of carbon dioxide, toxins, and tension held in the body and mind. Ideally, the exhalations should be about twice as long as the inhalations. Initially, if you count to five as you inhale and exhale, gradually try to make your exhalations to count of six, then seven, then eight, and so on until you feel more comfortable lengthening your exhalations.

The victorious breath—Ujjayi breath

Ujjayi, pronounced "oo-jai," is the joining of two Sanskrit root words, *uj* meaning "upward," and *jayi* meaning "victorious." Ujjayi helps the mind to rise beyond its typical state of restlessness and agitation to a calmer, more meditative state of clarity. It is a type of glottal breath which makes a distinctive sound that recalls the sound of the ocean and reminds us of the wave-like pattern of our breath. The glottis at the back of the throat is partially closed which narrows the passage of air to the trachea. It is recommended for use in all asana practice and, in many traditions, students are encouraged to maintain ujjayi breath at all times during asana practice. Once learned, it is a simple technique that can be practiced during nearly any activity, not just asana. It helps to relieve feelings of frustration and irritation, soothe a stressful mind. Consistent use of ujjayi increases consciousness of the breath and increases the ability to observe and learn more about the connection of mind, breath and body. We can go deeper into self-awareness and self-knowledge with the use of ujjayi.

To practice, first begin sitting in a comfortable spot, spine lengthened. Bring the shoulders up, back and down, away from the ears. Lift the heart and bow the head slightly. You can have the hands wherever they are comfortable or feel free to form jnana mudra (Figure 2.2, page 36) with each hand, palms facing upward. Take a slightly deeper inhalation than normal, expanding the belly. On the exhalation, constrict the glottis and the throat muscles slightly. The sound should remind you of Darth Vader's characteristic breath. Another way to get the sound is to pretend you are fogging up a mirror with your breath. Practice the "haaaahhh" sound with the mouth open and then gently close the mouth, maintaining the exhalation through the nostrils. The sound should remain. The breath itself is said to be a mantra, making the sound of the breath overt, it is the mantra *Hamsa*, which means, "I am that." The sound *ham* is the sound of each inhalation and the sound *sa* is the exhale. Ujjayi helps us to be aware of that mantra, allowing us to sink deeper into the awareness of the True Self.

Practice ujjayi with all asana to increase your breath awareness and mental focus, to move to a state of calm, and to increase the easefulness of postures. When running or cycling or doing any aerobic activity, ujjayi can increase respiratory efficiency. Ujjayi can be practiced anytime you notice you feel irritated, stressed or upset to feel soothed fairly quickly. The technique can also be used during meditation to help maintain focus on the breath. Once you have learned how to maintain ujjayi, it can also be paired with deergha swasam, the three-part breath.

Alternate nostril breathing—Nadi suddhi/ Nadi shodhana/Anuloma-viloma

nadi = channel *suddhi/shodhana* = purification
anuloma = with the grain *viloma* = against the grain

Known by several different names, the purpose of this breath is to purify the energetic channels of the body. Nadi suddhi also promotes relief of anxiety and helps to calm the mind and body. It is one of the most calming of the pranayamas. The alternate nostril technique helps balance prana in the ida and pingala nadis, energy channels which spiral around sushumna, the central channel which corresponds with our spinal cord. Ida and pingala correspond with the right and left nostrils. Breathing through each alternately helps to balance the flow of prana throughout the energy body.

To practice, form Vishnu mudra with your right hand (Figure 7.72). Stretching out the fingers of your right hand, fold in your index and middle fingers. You will use your extended thumb and ring fingers to alternately close off and release your right and left nostrils as you practice nadi suddhi.

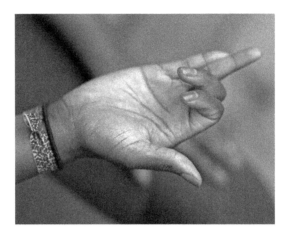

Figure 7.72 Vishnu mudra for practicing nadi suddhi breathing—the alternate nostril breath.

To practice, exhale fully and then inhale through both nostrils. Close off the right nostril with your thumb, and exhale slowly through the left. Inhale through the left. Release the thumb and close the left nostril with the ring finger. Exhale slowly through the right. Inhale through the right nostril, close it with the thumb. Release the left and exhale. Inhale through the left, close it. Release the right and exhale. Inhale through the right, close it. Continue this pattern (Figure 7.73).

You can use the nadi suddhi breath with the three-part breath of deergha swasam for an even deeper experience. Do this only if you practiced in the three-part breath as well as alternate nostril breathing.

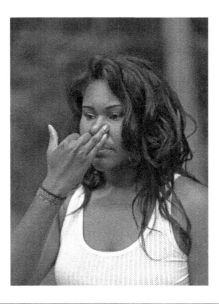

Figure 7.73 Practicing nadi suddhi breathing.

The skull shining breath—Kappalabhati

kappal=forehead, head, skull *bhati*=luminous, shining

Kappalabhati is a highly energizing breathing technique that is also a *kriya*, a yogic cleansing technique. It is said to heal problems of the sinuses, detoxify the lungs and also brings clarity of mind. The technique is also thought to benefit all the energy channels of the face, sinus cavity and the brain. In grief, this breath can help energize a grief-addled brain and body. It can help clean out toxins in the body which build up from poor eating habits, overuse of alcohol or other substances, and clear the sinuses which are often clogged from crying. The breathing pattern hyper-oxygenates the body and brain and lowers the levels of CO_2. It calms the respiratory system and relaxes the nervous system. The movement of the abdominal muscles and the exhalation of breath is similar to laughter and the breath increases endorphins, the "feel-good" hormones, in the brain. Those who have untreated high blood pressure, cardiac problems, seizure disorders or serious lung disorders are cautioned against practicing this pranayama.

This pranayama technique is rapid and employs a forceful, purposeful exhalation through the nose, while the inhalation is effortless and soundless. In practicing kappalabhati, we snap the abdomen in quickly while exhaling forcefully through the nose, the inhale follows naturally and passively. This pattern is the opposite of normal breathing where the inhale is the more active and exhale is passive. Some students can get confused and reverse breathe, so please be mindful of ensuring that you are forcefully exhaling, not forcefully inhaling. The best way to describe the forceful active exhalation in kappalabhati is to think of a gnat flying up your nose and the fast, nearly reflexive forceful exhalation you use to get it out as fast as possible. When you do this, notice that the abdomen pulls in quickly to force the air out of the nose. The inhalation flows in naturally and easily.

To practice kappalabhati, either kneel or sit in a comfortable cross-legged position or erect in a chair. The chest should be lifted and the spine long. The head should remain erect and, with the exception of the abdominal movements, the body should remain as still as possible throughout the practice. You may want to practice with a hand on the abdomen to feel the movement of the musculature. Be sure that the abdomen is snapping in and upward with the exhalation. Slowly begin to get used to the movement, about one breath per second, and gradually increase the speed of the exhalations to 2–3 exhalations per second. Start with 30 breaths and then relax, breathing normally. You may increase the rounds up to 60 expulsions per minute with an eventual goal of 120 expulsions per minute. Allow the face to be relaxed, the jaw unclenched and the brow unfurrowed. If you feel lightheaded or dizzy, stop immediately and allow the breath to go back to normal. If this is the case, it is likely you are placing too much emphasis on the inhalation. Allow the inhalation to be completely passive with no effort at all.

Chant

The word "chant" is from the Latin *cantare*, meaning "to sing." While there are differences in singing and chanting, both can be used to focus, uplift, connect spiritually, expand the heart and mind, and lead to a contemplative, meditative state of communion with the Divine. Chants are generally rhythmic phrases sung by the voice but, unlike songs, they are specific intonations of word and sound that carry and transmit particular vibrations. Chant is found in many different traditions including Christianity, Judaism, Islam, Hinduism, Buddhism, Shinto, Sufism, Native American traditions and many others. Chants serve many purposes and do many things. Some tell stories, some are repeated prayers, some serve the purpose of worship. Chanting is used to induce trance, quiet the mind, lift the spirit, energize the body and mourn the dead.

There are many reasons to chant. It's fun. It's the making of a joyful noise. It is creative and expressive. Using the body as an instrument of sound vibration connects us to all of creation. It lifts us up and connects us to something greater than ourselves. When we chant, we commune with the Divine, with nature and with our beloved dead. We are sending energetic waves out into the Universe that are ever-expanding, reaching into depths that we will never see with our eyes.

Mantra japa

Japa is the repetition of a mantra and, while legitimately its own branch of yoga, the chanting of mantra is a form of pranayama as well as a form of dhyana, concentration. A mantra is a particular sound vibration, some of which are *bija*, "seed" mantras, specific sacred syllables which have no direct translation, but which resonate with Divine energy. The sacred sound of Om is one of these, as well as the seed mantras that resonate with each chakra. Some mantras have meanings, some are names of God or phrases of holy text.

Mantra Japa is often used with a *mala*, a string of beads, similar to the Catholic rosary, used as a tool to help the practitioner chant her mantra a particular number of times. Malas usually contain 108 beads, a sacred number in the Vedic traditions. The mantra is usually said 108 times, or a derivative of 108. Some malas may have 27 beads, which are each counted four times. Making and chanting with your own mala is a helpful bhakti practice and the mala can be worn as reminder of your practice and also as a connection to your beloved dead.

In practicing mantra japa, any mantra which resonates with you can be used, it doesn't have to be Sanskrit. Whatever you find uplifting and peace inducing for mind and body is perfectly fine.

Regardless of what mantra is used, the intent, the remembrance and the repetition of the mantra bring the results. The benefits of chanting mantra regularly are many and include stress reduction in everyday life, a mental focus to which the thoughts can turn when we are distressed or anxious. It is a helpful tool for both dhyana and dharana and can lead to meditation and samadhi. Mantras are generally short and simple to remember.

The simple and powerful Om (Figure 7.74) is an ideal mantra in itself. Chanting the sound of Om is a pranayama exercise and a spiritually powerful act.

To chant Om: The sound of Om is said to consist of four syllables: Aw/Oo/Mm and the silent syllable where the breath comes into the body.

- To begin to chant, take a deep inhalation into the belly and allow the sound to rise from the diaphragm.

- The first syllable is A, pronounced "awe." Beginning the sound at the back of the throat, you should feel it in the solar plexus and the chest.

- The second syllable is U, pronounced "ooo." As the sound moves to the upper palate, you should feel the throat vibrating.

- The third syllable is M, pronounced, "mmm..." As you chant the sound "mmm," bring the teeth together so the vibration is felt in the face and head. When this happens, the pineal gland is also stimulated. In chanting "mmm," the sound is drawn out until it merges with the silence of the Infinite, the final syllable.

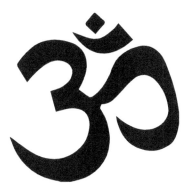

Figure 7.74 The symbol for Om.

Kirtan

Kirtan is a Hindu tradition of the call and response practice of chanting songs of praise and the names of God. It is a practice of meditation, breathwork and Bhakti love in one. The past several years have seen a growing awareness and practice of kirtan. Local kirtan groups meet together regularly in cities all over the world to chant, sing, worship and pray. Chanting workshops and kirtan concerts fill up with bliss seekers looking to share their love of chant, song, and a connection to each other and the Divine Source.

Kirtan is a spiritual experience, regardless of one's religious affiliation, or lack thereof. At a kirtan gathering, everyone sits on the floor. The audience is usually in close proximity to the musicians and the kirtan *wallah*, meaning leader. The wallah sings and chants the mantra and the audience chants it back. The mantras and the songs are based on ancient chants. The process is organic and one chant may go on for 30 minutes or longer. The energy is palpable. Each person has his or her own inner experience as well as with the collective group. Between chants, there may be long pauses of silence, movement of spirit and wordless communion with each other and with the Divine. Non-denominational and all inclusive, kirtan is for everyone.

Hari Om

This simple chant is a hello and hail to creation and Creator. Hari is pronounced "hah-ree" and means the name of God.

Hari Om, Hari Om, Hari Hari Hari Om

Hari Om, Hari Om, Hari Hari Om

Om Shanti—Om Peace

The sound of Om combined with Shanti, pronounced "shahn-tee," the Sanskrit word for Peace.

Om Shanti, Om Shanti, Om Shanti Om

Om Shanti, Om Shanti, Om Shanti Om

Om Purnamadah

The opening sloka, a peace prayer, from the *Ishvasya Upanishad* expresses our full completeness and connectedness both to one another and to the Source.

Om, purnamadah purnamidam purnaat purnamudachyate

purnasya purnaamadaya purnameva vashishyate

Om Shanti, Shanti, Shanti

This is whole, that is whole

When a portion of wholeness is removed,

that which remains is whole.

Om Peace, Peace, Peace.

Om Tryambakam

A healing mantra, the Om Tryambakam is also traditionally chanted at the crossing over and transitioning of a spirit after the death of the physical body.

Om tryambakam yajaamahe

Sugandim pushti vardhanam

Urvaa-rukamiva bandhanaan

Mrityor mokshya, ma'amritat

Om Shanti, Shanti, Shanti

We worship the All-seeing One
Fragrant, He nourishes bounteously,
From the fear of death may he set us free,
To realize immortality.
Om Peace, Peace, Peace

Om Asatoma

A prayer from the *Brihadaranyaka Upanishads* (1.3.28) which asks that ignorance of who we truly are be removed and that we be fully able to see the Truth of our eternal nature.

Om Asatoma sat gamaya
Tamasoma jyotir gamaya
Mrityor ma'am-ritam gamaya
Om Shanti, Shanti, Shanti

Lead us from unreal to real
Lead us from darkness to the light
Lead us from the fear of death to the knowledge of Immortality.
Om Peace, Peace, Peace

Sangha—Finding community

Sangha is the Sanskrit word for group or community. In grief we need our sangha. Finding your tribe, your group, your people is central to growth and a return to wholeness. Support in grief is a form of self-care. Those who are able to find good help and support are far better able to manage the pain of grief. Seek out those who are non-judgmental and compassionate; people who will not tell you what you should do, or shouldn't do, or what you need to do, or what you need to stop doing. Find a friend or family member who can be there for you. Attend a support group. Often local hospices have listings of support groups in local areas. Support groups can be very helpful for grieving people and can provide the kind of non-judgmental listening support grieving people need. Remember, though, that not all support groups are for all people. Find a place where you feel you belong.

Seek out online groups for your particular loss. Those who have shared similar losses can have an understanding that others cannot. Online communities can be extremely helpful sources of support in grief and life-long connections can be made.

You may want to explore the idea of seeking professional help with a trained grief counselor. Choosing a counselor or therapist is a very personal decision. The most important element in a therapeutic relationship is the relationship itself. If you trust the therapist and feel safe with him or her, this is the number one consideration. When deciding to work with a mental health professional, always ask about his or her experience in working with grief.

You may also want to seek out a yoga sangha as well as a grief sangha. Some lucky people may find both of those in one place. Not all yoga centers offer classes to support grief and loss, but some do. A gentle yoga class, restorative yoga, yin yoga or beginning classes are good places to start your yoga journey. If you are nearby an ashram or a yoga center, explore their workshops and attend one that sounds appealing to you. If you don't have access to specialty classes like yoga for grief, you might think about getting some of your grief sangha together to form a yoga circle and create practices together based on this book.

The most important thing is to honor your own experiences, your beloved dead in the ways you wish, and to be as awake and aware as possible. I hope this book has provided some helpful tools that can support you in your travels. My love and sincere wishes for your continued growth go with you on your journey.

Atha Yoganusasanam, sutra 1:1
Yoga is Now.

References and Further Reading

Avila, St. Teresa. 2007a. *Interior Castle.* (Ed. E.A. Peers, trans. Ed.) New York, NY: Dover Thrift Publishing.

Avila, St. Teresa. 2007b. *St. Teresa of Avila: Devotions, Prayers and Living Wisdom.* (Ed: M. Starr; trans. Ed.). Boulder, CO: Sounds True Inc.

Cacciatore, J. 2013. *Selah: An Invitation Toward Fully Inhabited Grief.* Sedona, AZ: MISS Foundation and Center for Loss and Trauma Publishers.

Carroll, C. & Carroll R. 2012. *Mudras of India: A Comprehensive Guide to the Hand Gestures of Yoga and Indian Dance.* London: Singing Dragon.

Corporation for National and Community Service. 2007. *The Health Benefits of Volunteering: A Review of Recent Research.* Retrieved from http://www.nationalservice.gov/pdf/07_0506_hbr.pdf on May 12, 2015.

Frankl, V.E. 1986. *The Doctor and the Soul: From Psychotherapy to Logotherapy* (3rd ed.), (R. Winston, C. Winston, trans.). New York, NY: Random House.

Frankl, V.E. 2006. *Man's Search for Meaning.* Boston, MA: Beacon Press.

Frawley, D. 2000. *Vedantic Meditation.* Berkeley, CA: North Atlantic Books.

Hollick, M. 2006. *The Science of Oneness: A Worldview for the 21st Century.* The Bothy, Deershot Lodge, Park Lane, Ropley, Hants, SO24 OBE, UK: O-Books, John Hunt Publishing.

Iyengar, B.K.S. 1988. *The Tree of Yoga.* Boston, MA: Shambala Press.

John of the Cross, St. 2002. *Dark Night of the Soul* (M. Starr trans.). New York, NY: Riverhead Books.

Jung, C.G. 1989. *Memories, Dreams and Reflections.* New York, NY: Random House Publications.

Jung, C.G. 1996. *The Psychology of Kundalini Yoga.* Princeton, NJ: Princeton University Press.

Jung, C.G. *Contributions to Analytical Psychology.* 2006. London: Hesperides Press.

Jung, C.G. *Psychology and Alchemy.* 1980. Princeton, NJ: Princeton University Press.

Kaelber, W.O. (1976). Tapas, birth, and spiritual rebirth in the Vedas. *History of Religions,* 15, 343–386.

Kaminoff, L. & Matthews, A. 2012. *Yoga Anatomy* (2nd ed.). Champaigne, IL: Human Kinetics.

Keen, S., Valley-Fox, A. 1989. *Your Mythic Journey: Finding Meaning in Your Life Through Writing and Storytelling.* New York, NY: St. Martin's Press.

Kempton, S. 2013. *Awakening Shakti: The Transformative Power of the Goddesses of Yoga.* Boulder, CO: Sounds True Inc.

Levine, S. 2009. *Trauma, Tragedy, Therapy: The Arts and Human Suffering*. London: Jessica Kingsley Publishers.

Levine, S. & Levine, O. 1989. *Who Dies? An Investigation of Conscious Living and Conscious Dying*. New York, NY: Anchor Books.

Lewis, C.S. 1996. *A Grief Observed*. New York, NY: HarperCollins Publishers.

Marchand, P. 2007. *The Yoga of Truth*. Rochester, VT: Destiny Books.

Musick, M.A. & Wilson, J. 2003. Volunteering and depression: The role of psychological and social resources in different age groups. *Social Science and Medicine*, 56, 259–269

Narada, St. *Narada's Way of Divine Love: The Bhakti Sutras*. (S. Prabhavananda trans. Ed.) Hollywood, CA: Vedanta Press.

Patanjali. 2002. *Yoga Sutras of Patanjali* (M. Stiles trans.). San Francisco, CA: Red Wheel/Weiser LLC.

Patanjali. 2003. *The Yoga Sutras of Patanjali* (S. Satchidananda trans. Ed). Yogaville, Buckingham, VA: Integral Yoga® Publications.

Prabhavananda, S. 2000. *Narada's Way of Divine Love*. Hollywood, CA: Vedanta Press.

Satchinada, S. (trans., ed.) 2000. *The Living Gita: The Complete Bhagavad Gita, A Commentary for Modern Readers*. Yogaville, Buckingham, VA: Integral Yoga Publications.

Schwartz, C., Meisenhelder, J.B., Ma, Y. & Reed, G. (2003). Altruistic social interest behaviors are associated with better mental health. *Psychosomatic Medicine*, 65, 778–785.

Rea, S. 2014. *Tending the Heart Fire*. Boulder, CO: Sounds True Inc.

Rumi, J. *The Illuminated Rumi*. (Barks C. trans.). New York, NY: Broadway Books.

Starr, M. 2012. *God of Love: A Guide to the Heart of Judaism, Christianity and Islam*. Rhinebeck, NY: Monkfish Book Publishing Company.

Stiles, M. 2011. *Tantra Yoga Secrets: Eighteen Transformational Lessons to Serenity, Radiance and Bliss*. San Francisco, CA. Red Wheel/Weiser LLC.

Stiles, M. 2000. *Structural Yoga Therapy*. San Francisco, CA. Red Wheel/Weiser LLC.

Vivekananda, S. 2013. *Bhakti Yoga: The Yoga of Love and Devotion*. Kolkata, India: Trio Process.

Weller, F. 2012. *Entering the Healing Ground: Grief, Ritual and the Soul of the World*. Santa Rose, CA: WisdomBridge Press.

Williamson, M.A. 1996. *Return to Love*. New York, NY: HarperCollins Publishers Inc.

Index